BARNES & NOBLE HEALTH BASICS™

Thyroid Disorders

By Lewis Vaughn

BARNES
&NOBLE
BOOKS
NEW YORK

For information, contact:
Barnes & Noble
122 Fifth Avenue
New York, NY 10011
212-633-4000

About the Author

Lewis Vaughn is the author, editor, or contributing writer of a number of books on health, fitness, and medicine. Dozens of his articles on health and medicine have appeared in newspapers, newsletters, and national magazines. He is also the former editor of the newsletter *Nutrition Forum* and the former executive editor of the medical journal *The Scientific Review of Alternative Medicine*.

About the Contributors

Portions of this work were reviewed by Stephen Possick, M.D. , and Marcy Adlersberg Cheifetz, M.D., Clinical Instructor, Yale University, and Clinical Endocrinologist, Waterbury Hospital, Waterbury, CT. The nutritional information was written by Mindy Hermann, R.D. The information about searching the Internet was edited by Matt Lake. The information about complementary therapies was written by Melanie Hulse.

Barbara J. Morgan Publisher
Barnes & Noble Basics

Barb Chintz Editorial Director
Barbara Rietschel Art Director
Wynn Madrigal Editor
Emily Seese Editorial Assistant
Della R. Mancuso Production Manager

Illustrations by Cynthia Saniewski

Table of Contents

Foreword

If you or a loved one has just been diagnosed with a thyroid disorder, the first thing you will want to know is how to manage the condition effectively. This is where Barnes & Noble Health Basics *Thyroid Disorders* comes in. Written with expert guidance from leading physicians, this informative book leads you to a deeper understanding of your symptoms and treatment.

No matter what type of thyroid condition you have, you'll find plenty of useful information on treatment, medication, nutrition, complementary therapies, searching the Internet, and putting together a health-care team. You'll also get the latest news on cutting-edge research and some wise advice on the role of stress and comfort in managing your health.

With all of these helpful insights at your fingertips, you'll be able to take control of your thyroid condition and become an advocate for your own health care. Remember: An informed patient is an empowered one. So read on to put yourself in the driver's seat when it comes to treating and managing your thyroid disorder.

Barb Chintz
Editorial Director
Barnes & Noble Health Basics Series

Getting the Diagnosis

Experiencing the symptoms
what's going on?

What does it feel like to have a thyroid disorder? You may feel tired and depressed. You may be asymptomatic (meaning you have no discernible symptoms). Or you might feel hyperactive and irritable or sluggish and moody. But since these symptoms are so similar to those of stress and depression, most people tend to ignore them and carry on. Over time, however, other symptoms may start to appear, such as sensitivity to cold or changes in weight and digestion. But again, these symptoms can come on so slowly and are so unalarming that many people don't bother about them. That is, until the symptoms worsen to the point where a visit to the doctor is in order. If this was your story, then, hopefully, your doctor listened carefully to your changing health issues and ordered a blood test to check the level of thyroid hormones in your blood. (Thyroid hormones help regulate your metabolism.)

In some cases, though, your doctor may not piece your symptoms together, especially if you don't fit the typical thyroid profile, which is a woman over the age of 35 with symptoms of fatigue. And so your doctor may not have ordered thyroid screening blood tests. The reason for a misdiagnosis is twofold. Most people don't pay the right kind of attention to their bodies, and so they don't know how to talk effectively to their doctors about their symptoms. Whenever an expert and a layperson talk there is often miscommunication. Think back to the time when your car was on the fritz. Remember how you tried to explain the clunk-clunk noise to your mechanic and how he looked at you quizzically? Well, sometimes, talking to your doctor about your symptoms is just as difficult. (For more on how to overcome this natural communication problem, see page 118.) This is especially true for thyroid problems because the symptoms come on so gradually that months can go by before you have a full-blown complaint. Moreover, some people have absolutely no symptoms at all.

What can you do about this communication gap? For starters, you need to know the symptoms that arise with thyroid disorders. Curiously, they fall into two main camps. One group of symptoms is caused by having too much thyroid activity, known as **hyperthyroidism**; the other group of symptoms is due to too little thyroid activity, called **hypothyroidism**. Having several of these symptoms does not mean that you have a thyroid disorder, but it does mean that you need to talk to your doctor about them. Here's a roundup of typical thyroid symptoms:

Common Symptoms of Thyroid Disorders

Hyperthyroidism (overactive thyroid)	Hypothyroidism (underactive thyroid)
Weight loss	Weight gain
Fast heartbeat	Slow heartbeat
Enlarged thyroid gland	Enlarged thyroid gland
High blood pressure	Hoarse voice
Muscle weakness	Puffy face
Exhaustion, fatigue	Exhaustion, fatigue
Nervousness	Intolerance to cold
Depression	Depression
Sleep problems	Sleep problems
Restlessness	High cholesterol
Trembling	Menstrual changes
Bulging eyes	Slowed speech
Frequent bowel movements	Constipation
Diarrhea	Numbness
Infertility	Poor memory
Skin, hair, and nail changes	Skin, hair, and nail changes

Your emotional symptoms
thyroid disorders can affect your emotional well-being

If you have thyroid trouble, you may or may not have also experienced psychological symptoms as well as physical ones. The good news is that in most cases the psychological symptoms are mild, and they usually disappear when your thyroid problem is treated. The bad news is that you may not realize that your mental health has anything to do with a thyroid dysfunction and ignore feelings of depression and anxiety, which often coexist with thyroid disease. Moreover, depression and anxiety can persist despite treatment for thyroid disease.

Common Symptoms of Thyroid Disorders

Hyperthyroidism *(overactive thyroid)*	**Hypothyroidism** *(underactive thyroid)*
Noticeable anxiety and excitability	Impaired memory
Mood swings, including bouts of crying	Slowing of mental processes
Irritability and impatience	Inability to concentrate
Sensitivity to noise	Loss of interest in normal activities
Sleeplessness	Confused thinking
Short attention span	Depression
	Loss of interest in sex
	Withdrawal from friends and family

Psychological symptoms may occur with both hypothyroidism and hyperthyroidism. And while these psychological symptoms can seem pretty generic (depression for hypothyroidism; anxiety and mania with hyperthyroidism), when they are coupled with just a few of the physical symptoms, such as irregular heartbeat; severe fatigue; dry, rough skin; muscle weakness; weight gain; and dry, thin hair, you can be pretty certain that trouble is afoot. If that is the case, then a thyroid screening blood test is in order.

FIRST PERSON INSIGHTS

It's not just a woman's disease

I was 50 years old but felt like I was 80. I was dead tired when I went to bed at night, and I was the same way when I woke up. I had difficulty concentrating at my job. I felt like I was in a fog. Even worse, I started to get really depressed—for no reason. Everything seemed to be going okay in the rest of my life, but I still had a very serious case of the blues. I had been in this predicament for about a month when I finally went to my doctor for help. I was fearing the worst. I was afraid that he would say that my problem was cancer, or diabetes, or some psychiatric problem. But he didn't jump to conclusions. He just ordered a few blood tests. Later he called me with the results: I was hypothyroid, a condition that could be cleared up by supplying my body with the thyroid hormones that it lacked. I was shocked because I thought thyroid disorders were a "woman's disease." All I had to do was take a pill once a day. Within two weeks I was back to my old self. My dark days of fatigue and depression seemed a million miles away.

—John K., Amherst, NY

Similarities to other disorders
ruling out other disorders

As your doctor gives you a physical and listens to your symptoms, he will be lining up all the possible disorders and diseases that match your symptoms. He will then start eliminating them one by one, until he settles on the disorder or disease that most likely explains your symptoms. It's as if your doctor were a detective sifting through a list of suspects, looking for clues that point to the culprit.

Your doctor will ask you some very specific questions to help with the "rule out" phase, including:

Is this a new type of symptom? Was the onset abrupt? Did you ever lose consciousness? Do the symptoms get worse over the course of a day? at night? Do you have any other medical conditions, such as cancer or infection? What medical disorders run in your family?

But because most thyroid symptoms come on so slowly, it can be hard to talk about them in any useful detail. Moreover, it becomes very easy for both doctor and patient to blame these gradual symptoms on very common conditions that also come on gradually, namely menopause and aging.

Another problem is that most thyroid symptoms are not "acute," meaning sharp or severe. For example, if you are hyperthyroid, your chief complaints will be feeling restless and being unable to sleep. Because these symptoms have no apparent cause, a busy doctor might pass these off as stress. If you are hypothyroid and feeling tired and blue, your doctor may assume you are depressed and advise you to seek therapy or perhaps prescribe an antidepressant. For these reasons alone, a thyroid disorder is often misdiagnosed. Be concerned if your doctor says, without adequate thyroid testing, that your symptoms are the result of menopause, aging, depression, or stress. Ask your doctor if your problems could be thyroid related. Then ask if you can have a thyroid screening test to be sure.

Why thyroid disorders are similar to stress: When your body reacts to stress, you usually experience some very distinct bodily changes: Your heart races to increase the flow of blood to the muscles; your breathing increases to get more oxygen to the brain so it stays alert; and your digestion shuts down in order to send energy to the muscles. These are just a few of the responses that are hard wired in your body to help it handle a stressful situation. Once the stress has passed, your body then returns to its normal restful state. But what happens if there are chronic zaps of the stress responses and the body never gets a chance to return to a restful state? Researchers think that chronic stress, the curse of the modern age, can *trigger* a number of illnesses, such as thyroid disease. The problem is that the symptoms of stress often mimic the symptoms of thyroid disorders, so it's easy to put the blame on stress instead of on the underlying disease that chronic stress may have kickstarted. For more on stress, see pages 102–103.

Why they are similar to depression: When you are depressed, your body goes through a number of very specific physical and emotional changes. Some signs of clinical depression are listlessness, sleep disturbances, and poor memory. These symptoms are due to a chemical imbalance in your brain. Alas, the symptoms of depression are quite similar to those of hypothyroidism. In fact, they are so similar that most psychiatric hospitals routinely do a thyroid blood test on new patients to rule out thyroid disorders. Again, a busy doctor may easily dismiss your symptoms as depression and send you on your way with a prescription for antidepressants. Since depression often coexists with thyroid disease, the antidepressants may help your mood, but they will not abate any other thyroid-related symptoms.

Why they are similar to menopause: There are many thyroid "symptoms" associated with menopause. They include mood swings, depression, and dry skin. Thyroid disorders can also cause menstrual irregularities similar to those of early menopause. For this reason, women going through menopause should have a TSH blood test (see pages 18–19).

Keeping a health journal
learning to listen to your body

But what if your symptoms of "stress" or "depression" don't seem to go away? If you are like most people, you try to ignore them until you no longer can and then go to the doctor (again) and hope he can "fix whatever it is." But in order to do that, you need to provide very useful information about what is going on inside your body. That means learning how to really pay attention to your symptoms.

One of the best ways to keep tabs on your symptoms is to write them down in a journal. By tracking them you will learn to pay attention to your body and understand what it is trying to tell you. Over time, this health journal will be an invaluable tool that will enable both you and your doctors to recognize patterns that point to the right disorder.

Once you are correctly diagnosed, your health journal will be very helpful to your recovery. How so? Treatment for either hypothyroidism or hyperthyroidism does not necessarily happen overnight. It sometimes takes time to determine the right dose of medication to ease your symptoms. By noting changes in your symptoms as you undergo treatment, you can plot the success of various treatments. A health journal is a powerful tool that can save you time and unnecessary suffering. It also does a wonderful job of reminding you that you, not your doctors, are in charge of your health.

Sample of a health journal

Get a three-ring binder and fill it with loose-leaf paper. Next, set aside a time every week to record how you feel. Keep it simple. Cover each major body system and identify any symptoms. Grade each symptom on a scale of 0 to 10, with 0 being nonexistent and 10 being a major concern. Your goal is to track the lessening or worsening of any symptoms. If you wish, make copies of the chart below and use it to find patterns to your symptoms.

DATE							
SYMPTOMS							
Headache							
Throat swelling							
Hoarseness							
Muscle weakness							
Diarrhea							
Constipation							
Cold intolerance							
Heat intolerance							
Trembling hands							
Poor appetite							
Ravenousness							
Feelings							
Upbeat							
Depressed							
Low energy							
High energy							
Sleep							
Insomnia							
Excessive sleep							

Seeing your doctor
what the thyroid does

If your symptoms are getting worse, your health journal will reflect this. Your notes on your symptoms will be very useful to share with your doctor. When you report consistently high levels of restlessness, diarrhea, and insomnia for over two to three weeks, a doctor will suspect a thyroid problem. (That is not the case if you say something vague like "I just feel anxious. Oh, and my appetite is off.")

If your doctor suspects a thyroid problem, one of the first things she will do during your exam is to gently **palpate** (feel around with her fingers) your neck and throat. Your doctor is looking for any bulges or bumps in your neck to suggest that your thyroid is enlarged. (In fact, if you can easily feel your thyroid gland or feel a lump in that area, or you feel a fullness in your throat, you should see your doctor to have it checked out. Your thyroid could be enlarged, indicating that something may be wrong with it.)

Beneath the skin in the front of your neck, just below your larynx (voice box), rests your thyroid, a two-inch-wide gland shaped like a bow tie, shown here in blue.

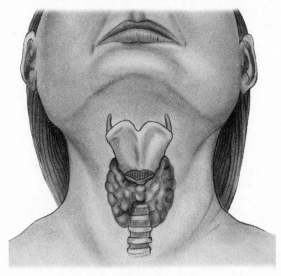

Why all the concern about an enlarged thyroid? The thyroid is a little gland with big responsibilities. It produces thyroid hormones that are released into your bloodstream to control your body's metabolism (the speed of your body's chemical processes), which influences nearly every cell and organ in your body.

When this gland malfunctions, the result is too little or too much thyroid hormone, which in turn can drastically change your body weight, energy level, skin condition, cholesterol level, muscle strength, mental alertness, mood, and more. Too much thyroid hormone in your bloodstream will speed up your metabolism, making cells and organs work faster. When the thyroid is overactive and produces too much hormone, **hyperthyroidism** is the result. Too little hormone slows everything down. When the thyroid is underactive and produces too little hormone, **hypothyroidism** occurs.

What keeps the thyroid in check? The thyroid is regulated by the pituitary gland, the undisputed master gland of the human body. The pituitary gland is buried deep inside the brain. It tells the thyroid how much thyroid hormone to produce, communicating its orders by manufacturing **thyroid-stimulating hormone,** or **TSH**. When the pituitary gland senses that there is too much thyroid hormone circulating in the blood, it releases less TSH. This tells the thyroid to calm down and release less hormone. Conversely, if there is too little thyroid hormone in your system, the pituitary releases more TSH, which revs up the thyroid to produce more hormone.

The pituitary's TSH stimulates the thyroid to make two very important hormones, called simply T_4 and T_3. To make these hormones, your thyroid needs iodine, which it gets from your diet (many foods contain iodine). Here's an important fact to remember: Your thyroid is the only thing in your whole body that needs iodine to work. If you don't have enough iodine in your diet, your thyroid will compensate by enlarging in size. (This is not a problem in North America because the diet is rich in foods that contain iodine, namely iodized salt, shellfish and certain vegetables.)

Thyroid blood tests
how doctors come to a diagnosis

If your doctor suspects thyroid trouble either from palpating your thyroid or from your symptoms, she will first order a blood test to track the amount of thyroid hormone in your blood. This is called the TSH blood test. Remember, TSH (thyroid-stimulating hormone) is produced by the pituitary gland and is an excellent indicator of thyroid-hormone levels. High TSH levels mean that your thyroid isn't making enough thyroid hormone and needs to make more; low TSH levels mean your thyroid is being told to cut back on hormone production (because your thyroid levels are too high). So if you are hyperthyroid (that is, you have elevated thyroid hormone levels), your TSH levels will be low. If you are hypothyroid, your TSH levels will be high.

The TSH test is extremely sensitive. It can pick up on hypothyroidism long before thyroid-hormone levels plummet. It can detect hyperthyroidism even when the disorder is in its early stages. Even better news is that the TSH blood test is also an excellent tool to help doctors monitor progress in your treatment. Once treatment starts, they use periodic TSH testing to ensure that you are getting the right amount of hormone. (For more on treatment and medication see pages 45–64.)

Doctors also use blood tests that directly measure the amount of the two key thyroid hormones in your system: T_4 and T_3. One such test is the so-called FT_4, which measures the amount of free-floating T_4 thyroid hormone in your bloodstream. Like the TSH test, the FT_4 can give your doctor some idea of how your thyroid is working. In unclear cases, a test called the FT_3 may be used to measure the amount of free-floating T_3 hormone in your system. Doctors may also test for **thyroid antibodies** in your blood. These cells signal the presence of an autoimmune disorder that can affect the thyroid. (See page 32 for more information on autoimmune thyroid diseases.)

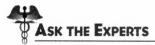

My TSH came back normal, so my doctor ruled out any thyroid problems. But my symptoms persist. What should I do?

Your symptoms, while similar to thyroid disorders, can actually be caused by other disorders, such as clinical depression or irritable bowel syndrome (a chronic disorder that results in fatigue and diarrhea). If you do feel that your health is not what it used to be, ask your doctor about these disorders.

I heard from my doctor that the guidelines for the TSH blood test have just been changed. Should I be retested?

In 2003 the American Association of Clinical Endocrinologists narrowed the range for the amount of TSH in the blood. The new guidelines say normal should be between 0.3 and 3.0 mlU/L (micro units per milliliter of blood). Previously, normal was anything between 0.5 and 5.0 mlU/L. These new guidelines mean that a lot more people will be diagnosed with thyroid disorders in the future. If your old test scores are outside the norm of the new guidelines, see your doctor and get retested.

Can you ever get false readings in a thyroid blood test?

Yes. If you are taking certain medications, they can affect your thyroid levels, thereby altering your thyroid tests—although, typically, your thyroid function test should remain normal. The main drug culprits are aspirin, heparin (a blood-thinning drug), furosemide (a diuretic), diphenylhydantoin (an anticonvulsant drug), and orphenadrine citrate (a muscle relaxant). Before you take a thyroid test, be sure to tell your doctor which over-the-counter or prescription medication you are taking. Pregnancy can affect TSH levels, as can birth control pills. Be sure to tell your doctor if you are pregnant or taking any medication.

Thyroid scans
how doctors come to a diagnosis

The TSH tests will indicate only that you have a thyroid problem. They will not show how severe the problem is or what caused it. Other tests can. An important one is the **radioactive iodine uptake test (RAI)**. In an uptake test, you are given a tiny amount of radioactive iodine in capsule form. Since the only cells in your body that use iodine are thyroid cells, doctors can test how much or how little of the radioactive iodine your thyroid uses. After taking the special pill, you will be sent home for 6 to 24 hours—enough time for the radioactive iodine to collect in your thyroid gland. You will return to the lab and a counter will be placed over your neck to measure how much radioactive iodine has been absorbed by your thyroid. A high absorption, or uptake, of radioactive iodine means that your thyroid is producing too much of the thyroid hormones, T_3 and T_4. A low absorption means your thyroid is not taking up iodine, which can be caused by several things. In most cases, it usually indicates thyroiditis, an inflammation of the thyroid (see page 40) that is often accompanied by hyperthyroidism.

In some cases, the lab will also do a scan of your neck after a radioactive uptake test. This is called a **thyroid scan**. Doctors will request this X-ray if you have any lumps or nodules on your thyroid. The radioactive scan will show if the lumps are active, or "hot," and making thyroid hormone or "cold" and not making any thyroid hormone. The scan can also reveal the size of the thyroid and if it has grown. For more on bumps and growths, see pages 22–23.

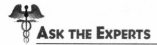

ASK THE EXPERTS

Do thyroid scans hurt?

They are virtually painless. The most uncomfortable part is having to remain still during the imaging process and having to hold your neck in an awkward position. If you get an injection during the procedure, you may feel a slight pinch.

I'm worried that the radioactive iodine used in a thyroid scan will cause cancer.

When testing, lab technicians only use a type of radioactive isotope that has a very short half-life, meaning it will be expelled from your body in a short time. There is no increased risk of cancer from having an uptake test. Pregnant or nursing women, however, should not have radioactive iodine uptake tests. Every kind of medical test is associated with at least some risk, no matter how small. So the important question is whether the risks of the test outweigh the benefits. In the case of thyroid testing, experts agree that for most people the benefits far outweigh the risks.

What if I'm allergic to shellfish?

People who are allergic to shellfish (which contain iodine) should tell their doctor of their allergy. The amount of iodine in the uptake test is so tiny that it is unlikely to cause any allergic reaction.

How accurate is the thyroid scan?

These tests have an accuracy rating of 80 to 85 percent, meaning that 80 to 85 percent of the time the tests give an accurate picture of your thyroid's condition. Sometimes, though, more than one thyroid test is given to confirm earlier results or to gather additional information.

Tests for bumps and lumps
how doctors come to a diagnosis

Sometimes your thyroid will try to solve its hormonal imbalance on its own. How? Again, remember that the thyroid is the only organ in your body that needs iodine to make its thyroid hormone. If you don't have enough iodine in your diet, your thyroid will compensate by enlarging in size. This makes sense when you think about it. The bigger your thyroid gets, the more cells it then has to grab more iodine, so it can make more thyroid hormone. When the thyroid grows an expanding mass, doctors call it a **goiter**. Goiters are not usually a problem in the U.S. because the average diet contains all the iodine you need. (Note: Some table salt has iodine added to it. Sea salt and kosher salt do not.)

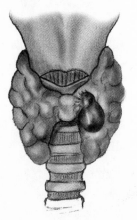

A cyst, or a lump (also known as a nodule, shown at left in blue), on the thyroid can also occur for a variety of other reasons. For the most part, these extra thyroid growths are benign (non-cancerous). But a small percentage can be cancerous, which is why your doctor will need to test them.

If your doctor finds a growth, chances are he will order a fine-needle aspiration (FNA). In this test, a super-thin hypodermic needle is inserted into the lump. This procedure is fairly painless—doctors usually numb the area first. A tissue sample is then extracted from the lump and examined under a microscope. This test can tell your doctor what's going on inside your thyroid and whether the cells in the lump are benign or malignant (cancerous). For more on thyroid cancer, see pages 65–80.

Doing the "Neck Check"

Doctors aren't the only ones who can look for signs of thyroid trouble. You can do a simple self-exam of your neck to see if your thyroid looks and feels normal. If it does not pass this test, you may need to have your doctor check it out. The American Association of Clinical Endocrinologists (AACE) has come up with a technique for doing a quick and easy inspection of your thyroid. The AACE calls it the "Neck Check." To do it, all you need is a glass of water and a small mirror.

1. Hold the mirror in your hand, focusing on the area of your neck just below the Adam's apple and immediately above the collarbone. Your thyroid is located in this area of your neck.

2. While focusing on this area in the mirror, tip your head back.

3. Take a drink of water and swallow.

4. As you swallow, look at your neck. Check for any bulges or protrusions in this area when you swallow. Reminder: Don't confuse the Adam's apple with the thyroid gland. The thyroid gland is located farther down on your neck, closer to the collarbone. You may need to repeat this process several times.

5. If you do see any bulges or protrusions in this area, see your physician. You may have an enlarged thyroid gland or a thyroid nodule and should be checked to determine whether cancer is present or whether treatment for thyroid disease is needed.

Getting the diagnosis
the good news and the bad

The test results are in. You are asked to come back to see the doctor. He tells you that your test results show a thyroid disorder and he will give you the name of the disease that is causing your symptoms and outline your treatment. Finally, your health puzzle is solved. You now have a name to put to your symptoms.

If your symptoms are hyperthyroid (weight loss, restlessness, bulging eyes, and so on) and your thyroid tests reveal too much thyroid hormone and the presence of thyroid antibodies, you may be told you have **Graves' disease**, an autoimmune disorder that attacks the thyroid (see page 34). In autoimmune diseases, cells in the body that normally protect it from illness or infection start to attack it. Graves' disease may also lead to both eye and skin diseases. **Thyroid eye disease,** or TED, accounts for the bulging, redness, and grainy feeling in the eyes. **Thyroid skin disease** brings with it a thickening or redness of the skin (especially on the shins). Hopefully, these symptoms will be controllable when the underlying hyperthyroidism is treated.

Another cause of hyperthyroidism is **thyroiditis,** an inflammation of the thyroid gland (see page 40). The inflammation is usually caused by an infection. While it usually goes away on its own, it can lead to permanent thyroid problems.

Sometimes **nodules** (or lumps) form on the thyroid gland. Over time these lumps can essentially become minithyroid glands. They can produce the thyroid hormones (T4 and T3), just as the thyroid itself does. Soon there is much more thyroid hormone circulating than the body needs, and hyperthyroidism is the result.

If your test results show too little thyroid hormone and thyroid antibodies, your doctor may suspect an autoimmune disease called **Hashimoto's**

thyroiditis (see page 38). It is the cause of the most common kind of thyroid inflammation. In Hashimoto's, as in Graves', disease, certain cells in the body attack the thyroid gland. Specifically, white blood cells and other antibodies strike thyroid cells, knocking many of them out of action. Without a full complement of thyroid cells, the thyroid cannot produce enough thyroid hormone, and hypothyroidism is the result. Sometimes people who have Hashimoto's thyroiditis have enlarged thyroids (goiters).

Autoimmune diseases? Inflammation of the thyroid? This all sounds pretty serious. Especially when your doctor explains that while your thyroid problem is easily treatable, there is no known cure. For some it may be a relief to have a name on which to hang their symptoms; for others it can be upsetting to hear that they now have a chronic illness.

The shock of getting a diagnosis

Everyone reacts differently when they are diagnosed with a chronic disorder. If your symptoms were nominal, then the common reaction is surprise and an immediate focus on treatment. For many people, it's a nonissue. They take a pill a day and don't think about it. But for those who have been plagued with uncomfortable symptoms for more than a few months, there can be a whole host of feelings, from fear and anger to sadness and resignation. Being associated with a named disease can be disconcerting because it changes your status quo. Having a named illness can sometimes even trigger the stress response in which blood rushes to the muscles, which can sometimes fog the brain; for more on this see pages 150–152. This could explain why so many people cannot take in what their doctor is saying when they get their diagnosis. The shock of hearing their diagnosis can trigger the stress response: Their bodies tense, their hearts race, and their minds sometimes freeze. Oftentimes, it's only when they get home that the news sinks in.

Possible causes

why you, why now?

One of the unsolved mysteries about thyroid disorders is what exactly causes them, especially such autoimmune conditions as Graves' disease and Hashimoto's thyroiditis. Doctors have known for more than a century that thyroid dysfunction is due to the overabundance or lack of various thyroid hormones, but they are still adding to the list of things that cause hormone production to go haywire.

In a world that is becoming increasingly industrialized and complex, more and more of these hidden culprits are turning out to be environmental. The use of chemicals (especially pesticides) in food production is now implicated in many autoimmune diseases. When the body goes into overdrive to protect itself against these chemical assailants, it produces too many antibodies, which can trigger Hashimoto's or Graves' disease.

Ironically, new findings also reveal that some of the nutritional aids we use to try to live healthier lives, such as kelp and soy products, can cause thyroid problems. Kelp contains concentrated amounts of iodine, and excess iodine can lead to hyperthyroidism. Soy products contain high amounts of soy isoflavones, which are hormones that behave much like estrogen. One theory purports that the overuse of soy products (and, likewise, estrogen supplements) is behind the rising rates of infertility and other endocrine problems, including thyroid dysfunction.

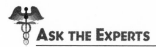

ASK THE EXPERTS

I've just been diagnosed with Graves' disease. I also suffer from fibromyalgia. Could one have caused the other?

When it comes to determining the causes of autoimmune disorders, such as Graves' disease or Hashimoto's thyroiditis, it is very difficult to pinpoint a cause. A great many health disorders will weaken the immune system, so it's possible, though not likely, that having fibromyalgia triggered your thyroid disorder. Conversely, huge swings in your thyroid levels could trigger fibromyalgia. The relationship between the endocrine system and the immune system is very complex. For more on advances in immunity, see pages 208–209.

I was diagnosed with depression last year and have been on antidepressants. They helped beat the depression, but I recently discovered that I have a thyroid disorder. Did my depression cause it?

That's a tough one. Researchers know there is a link between depression and some thyroid disorders. Thyroid disease can cause depression. Conversely, depression can cause abnormalities in thyroid function tests; these function tests usually return to normal with treatment for the depression. The good news is that there is treatment for both disorders.

You and the big picture
you're not alone

It's natural to ask, "Why me?" Chances are there are some risk factors that you have that make you more likely to have a thyroid problem. For example, those with a family history of thyroid disorders are more likely to have thyroid problems themselves. Women are up to eight times more likely than men to be afflicted with a thyroid disorder. This is why some people dub it a "woman's disease." The elderly also have an especially large share of thyroid problems. By age 60, 17 percent of women and 9 percent of men will be affected with thyroid disorder.

Is Prevention Possible?

If thyroid disorders run in your family, it makes sense to ask about prevention. Doctors are often asked if there are any natural supplements people can take now to head off thyroid problems in the future. This question is the subject of much debate. Attempting to lessen thyroid problems by self-dosing with kelp or organic iodine, for example, can backfire and result in hyperthyroidism. The best prevention is knowledge. Be sure to have your thyroid tested every five years after the age of 35, especially if thyroid disease runs in your family. Those over 60 should have their thyroid checked annually.

There are some preventive steps you can take now, however. In general, it is a good idea to stick to a low-fat, low-carbohydrate diet and take a multivitamin-multimineral supplement that emphasizes the antioxidant vitamins (A, C, E, and all the B's) and the mineral selenium. These natural antioxidants help to neutralize toxic substances in the body. This is crucial for maintaining adequate thyroid-hormone levels and keeping your thyroid gland healthy. Recent research also suggests that consuming too many soy products, such as tofu and soy milk, can lead to thyroid problems, so you might want to limit your intake of those products.

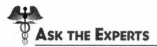

Several members of my family have experienced thyroid problems. Does this family trend indicate that I am destined to have a thyroid disorder?

No! But having a long family history of thyroid disease does suggest that you have an increased risk of getting the disease yourself. Also, the prevalence of certain other diseases or conditions in your family tree may indicate that thyroid trouble runs in your family and that you are therefore at a higher risk of developing thyroid problems. These conditions include hair loss, premature graying, and vitiligo (a skin condition that depletes pigmentation). If you suspect that thyroid disorders run in your family, you should alert your doctor, get a thyroid test, and urge the rest of your family to do the same. According to thyroid experts, even people who don't have a history of thyroid problems or don't suspect any should have their thyroid tested every five years starting at age 35.

Doesn't having enough salt in my diet offset the chances of my ever getting thyroid trouble?

Iodine is the one element the body needs to create thyroid hormone. Your body extracts it from the food that you eat. Usually, people in North America get all the iodine they need from their diet. This intake of iodine is due in large part to the practice of adding iodine to salt. (Thus the term *iodized salt*.) In Third World countries, however, iodine deficiency is widespread, resulting in 200 million people with goiters. Because iodine is so readily available in a typical North American diet, taking iodine supplements is not recommended. Those who do supplement their iodine risk getting an overdose of the element.

Helpful resources

The Chronic Illness Workbook
by Patricia Fennell

The Thyroid Sourcebook
by M. Sara Rosenthal

Thyroid Disease: The Facts
by R.I.S. Bayliss and
W.M.G. Tunbridge

**Thyroid Foundation of America,
Inc.**
Tel: 800 832-8321
Fax: 617 534-1515
www.allthyroid.org

**American Foundation of Thyroid
Patients**
Tel: 432 694-9966
www.thyroidfoundation.org

*Merck Manual of Medical
Information*
www.merck.com

Gland Central
(Internet source of thyroid
information)
www.glandcentral.com

CHAPTER 2

Types of Thyroid Disorders

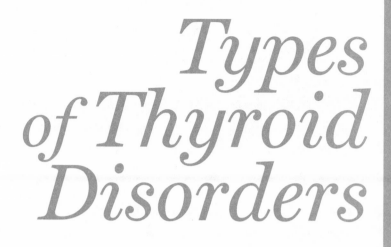

Thyroid disorders in a nutshell
the three main problems

Your thyroid is supposed to release just the right measure of thyroid hormone for your needs. But sometimes things go wrong and problems ensue. When it comes to your thyroid, these problems fall into three major categories: autoimmune disorders, inflammation of the thyroid, and structural problems with the thyroid. (Your problem can also be a combination of two or all three.) What's unusual about thyroid disorders is that they may cover the entire range of thyroid symptoms. In other words, you can start out with hyperthyroid (overactive thyroid) symptoms and end up with hypothyroid (underactive thyroid) symptoms. But you may have no symptoms at all.

Autoimmune disorders

The vast majority of all thyroid disorders are due to two distinct autoimmune diseases. Yes, that can sound scary, but actually autoimmune disorders are more common than you realize. Normally, when the body is under attack from a virus or an infection, it issues antibodies to kill off these foreign invaders. In an autoimmune disease, the body gets confused and cannot tell foreign cells from normal cells. The result? The body attacks its own normal cells in an attempt to stay healthy, when, in fact, it is doing much damage. Usually, autoimmune disorders target a particular part of the body; for example, in rheumatoid arthritis the body's joints are attacked.

One of the two autoimmune diseases that strike the thyroid is called Graves' disease; the other is called Hashimoto's disease. In Graves' disease, the body's defense cells attack the thyroid and cause it to produce too much thyroid hormone. In Hashimoto's disease, the body's antibodies attack the thyroid and, in effect, disable it. The result is too little thyroid hormone. While researchers do not know yet why these two different autoimmune diseases attack the thyroid, they do know that your chances of getting one of them are much more likely if anyone in your family has had one.

Inflammation

Another type of thyroid disorder occurs when the thyroid becomes inflamed. In medicine, any inflammation ends in *"itis,"*—for example, tendinitis or bronchitis. The same goes for the thyroid. Hence, the name **thyroiditis.** There are three types of thyroiditis—one is painful, the other two are not. The painful one is called **subacute thyroiditis.** It is usually caused by a virus and is "self-limiting" (in other words, it will go away on its own). The two painless ones are **silent thyroiditis** and **postpartum thyroiditis.** They are both caused by an autoimmune malfunction similar to that of Hashimoto's. They usually resolve on their own, but they can sometimes lead to permanent hypothyroidism. Unfortunately, the hypothyroid symptoms of postpartum thyroiditis mimic the postpartum "baby blues," so few women seek treatment for it. The good news is that after a few months the thyroid usually returns to normal. In about 5 to 10 percent of the postpartum cases, however, it does not and medical treatment is needed.

Growths

There is yet another type of problem that can impact the health of the thyroid and upset its delicate hormone activity. These are various growths and tumors on the thyroid that can impair its structural integrity. Doctors have different names for these growths, depending on their characteristics. They can be called goiters, nodules, or cysts. In the vast majority of cases, thyroid growths are benign, and at the most they can affect the production of thyroid hormone. But in rare cases these growths can be cancerous. This is why a doctor will want to do a test on a growth (see page 22) to determine which type it is.

Once your thyroid disorder has been diagnosed, your doctor has an amazing arsenal of treatment options. Alas, while there is no "cure" for any of these thyroid disorders, there are plenty of treatments available to mitigate the symptoms (see Chapter 3 for more on this).

Graves' disease
a common hyperthyroid disorder

Why does a perfectly normal thyroid slip into overdrive? In 70 to 80 percent of overactive-thyroid cases, the cause is Graves' disease. This is an autoimmune disorder in which the body's immune system fools the thyroid into manufacturing too much thyroid hormone. (The disease is named for the doctor Robert Graves, who first diagnosed it back in the 19th century.) Too much thyroid hormone results in hyperthyroid symptoms: fast and irregular heartbeat, shakiness, warm and moist hands, increased sweating, nervousness, increased appetite, high blood pressure, eye changes causing an intense stare, weight loss, diarrhea, intolerance to heat, muscle weakness, sexual dysfunction, exhaustion, and sleeplessness.

Thyroid experts are fairly certain that Graves' disease, the most prevalent form of hyperthyroidism, arises from a defect in the immune system. The normal job of the immune cells known as lymphocytes is to produce antibodies that help protect against viruses, cancer cells, and other enemies of the body. But some people (up to 10 percent of the population) produce antibodies that harm the body's own tissues. Sometimes these antibodies attack thyroid cells, stimulating them to overproduce thyroid hormone, ushering in hyperthyroidism (especially Graves' disease) along with a goiter (enlarged thyroid). The presence of hyperthyroidism, goiter, and eye disease together secure the diagnosis.

Some thyroid experts think that this autoimmune chain reaction is triggered by severe emotional stress, such as the death of a loved one or loss of a job. One theory is that stressful events cause an increase in levels of stress hormones, such as adrenaline, which then jump-start antibody production in the immune system. Whatever the case, it is complex, because many who get Graves' disease seem to have no major causes of stress in their lives.

Graves' disease is many times more likely to occur in women (especially those between 20 and 40) than in men. For reasons that doctors don't yet understand, Graves' disease also runs in families, though it's not clear whether Graves' is hereditary (due to a defective gene) or caused by something else that is common to family members, such as a viral infection. (A viral infection may explain why both George and Barbara Bush developed Graves' disease during his presidency.)

Once Graves' disease is diagnosed, treatment is fairly straightforward. Thyroid medication, radioactive iodine, and surgery are the basic options (see pages 45–64). In most people, these treatments are very effective at curing or controlling the disease. With these treatments, people feel well again in three months to a year, depending on the type of treatment. The downside is that even if treatment is a success, people will most likely develop symptoms of hypothyroidism someday. That's because thyroid treatments for Graves' often damage the thyroid, which leads to symptoms of hypothyroidism. Synthetic thyroid hormone can easily rectify this situation (see pages 54–57).

Thyroid eye disease
the reason behind the bulging eyes

Most cases of hyperthyroidism are caused by Graves' disease, and most symptoms of hyperthyroidism and Graves' disease are the same. One symptom in particular is the bulging, staring eyes—the classic look of hyperthyroidism. The stare occurs because the eyelids retract a bit, exposing a larger portion of the whites and creating the wide-eyed appearance. But sometimes people with Graves' disease develop a particular type of severe eye trouble known as thyroid eye disease, or TED. It's also known as Graves' ophthalmopathy. Here the eyes not only bulge, but the muscles of the eyeball may be affected too, possibly causing blurred or double vision. The inflammation can also make your eyes look red and watery and feel gritty and painful. Occasionally, the eyes are not watery at all, but very dry. If you have TED and you look in the mirror, you may observe more than just staring or bulging eyes. You may see bags under your eyes or puffiness around them, and the corners may be bloodshot.

TED arrives in stages and can begin months before the other symptoms of Graves' disease show up. The severity of TED symptoms can also vary dramatically. Some people may not be aware that they have eye problems because the symptoms are so mild. Very often, when the hyperthyroidism is treated, the TED symptoms go away. A few people, though, may be left with some permanent damage.

It's easy for your physician to overlook TED or mistake it for some other disorder. She may legitimately wonder: Is it conjunctivitis (pinkeye)? Is it allergies? Is it some other type of eye infection? The only way to know for sure is to have your thyroid tested.

Watch Out for a Thyroid Storm

In rare cases, hyperthyroidism can be more than a challenging disorder; it can be a good reason to call 911. This condition is known as thyroid storm. It's the result of an overload of thyroid hormone. It can occur when hyperthyroidism is left untreated for a long period or it can follow an infection. People in a thyroid storm can have an erratic or rapid heartbeat, high blood pressure, vomiting, diarrhea, high temperature, shock, even heart failure. If it is not treated right away, it can be fatal. Fortunately, thyroid storm is rare nowadays because hyperthyroidism is usually detected and treated before it gets out of control.

FIRST PERSON INSIGHTS

Don't light up

I knew smoking was bad for your heart and lungs. But who knew it was bad for your thyroid? I didn't until I was diagnosed with thyroid eye disease. Graves' disease runs in my family. Unfortunately, smokers who get Graves' disease are almost certain to also get thyroid eye disease. I so wish I had known there was such a strong connection between smoking and TED. I would have quit a whole lot sooner.

—Maggie T., Durham, NC

Hashimoto's thyroiditis
another common autoimmune disorder

Why does a perfectly normal thyroid slip into decline? There are a number of reasons, one of them an autoimmune disorder called Hashimoto's disease—so named for the Japanese surgeon who first discovered it back in 1912. Hashimoto's disease is common in elderly women and will probably occur in 10 percent of all women during their lifetime. Again, the cause is unknown, but doctors do see a genetic component, which means that if anyone in your family has had Hashimoto's you have a greater risk of getting it. Typically, you have no symptoms. This disease is usually discovered during routine blood tests.

In Hashimoto's disease, the lymphocytes (white blood cells that are part of the body's immune system) bombard the thyroid gland. This attack causes inflammation in the gland, which can lead to a painless goiter or a growth on the neck. It may take years, but ultimately the thyroid antibodies will cause the thyroid to shut down. How long will it be before you feel any effects of the disease? The speed at which Hashimoto's thyroiditis turns into full-blown hypothyroidism is apparently linked to the levels of Hashimoto's antibodies and TSH in your blood. This means that people with larger amounts of antibodies or TSH can experience the symptoms of hypothyroidism sooner than women who have lower levels. Research suggests that this transition to thyroid underactivity is much faster in women who are 45 and older.

Doctors base their diagnosis on thyroid function tests, such as the TSH blood test. The presence of antibodies in the blood will further confirm that the hypothyroidism is due to Hashimoto's disease.

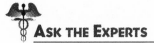

Ask the Experts

Can Hashimoto's thyroiditis lead to hyperthyroidism as well as hypothyroidism?

Yes. Sometimes the assault on thyroid cells forces thyroid hormones out of the thyroid and into the bloodstream, causing a brief episode of hyperthyroidism. This is called Hashitoxicosis. It can last for several weeks up to a few months. But soon the thyroid stops functioning altogether and hypothyroidism sets in.

Does Hashimoto's thyroiditis cause lumps on the thyroid gland?

Sometimes. Your thyroid may enlarge because of the inflammation that comes with Hashimoto's and feel lumpy in texture upon examination. If lumps do appear on your thyroid while you have Hashimoto's, you should have your physician check them to ensure that they are not an indication of cancer.

Is it possible to have other autoimmune diseases along with Hashimoto's thyroiditis?

Yes. Some people with Hashimoto's also have autoimmune disorders such as pernicious anemia, Sjögren's syndrome, lupus, celiac disease, and rheumatoid arthritis. They can also have endocrine disorders, such as diabetes and an underactive adrenal gland.

Thyroiditis
an inflamed thyroid

Certain kinds of illnesses can cause an inflammation of the thyroid, other-wise known as thyroiditis. The good news is that most of the illnesses that can inflame the thyroid are short-lived and do little damage.

Subacute granulomatous thyroiditis

This disorder begins as a common viral infection, such as a cold, and then spreads to the thyroid gland, where inflammation sets in, causing pain, fever, and tenderness in the neck. Thyroid hormone spills out into the bloodstream, instigating hyperthyroidism. Fortunately, this overactive phase is usually brief, from a few days to five or six weeks. Thyroid function soon returns to normal, then becomes underactive for a while, and finally goes back to normal. Most of the time, no permanent damage is done to the thyroid gland. Rarely, though, this disease can return and cause permanent hypothyroidism, which must be treated.

Silent lymphocytic thyroiditis

Silent lymphocytic thyroiditis (or painless thyroiditis) is like subacute thyroiditis except that the condition is usually painless and symptomless even though the thyroid is enlarged. For several weeks or months, mild hyperthyroidism is present, followed by mild hypothyroidism. Then thyroid function goes back to normal. Generally, people with silent thyroiditis are completely unaware of their condition. The only worrisome aspect of silent thyroiditis is that about 10 percent of those who have it may end up with permanent hypothyroidism, which requires treatment.

This disorder occurs mostly in women after giving birth (see pages 178–179) and is one of the thyroid disorders included in the more general term **postpartum thyroiditis**. Postpartum thyroiditis happens in up to 10 percent of women who give birth, usually a few months after delivery. Many women experience depression after pregnancy, and postpartum thyroiditis is often the cause. Women who develop postpartum thyroiditis are at an increased risk of permanent hypothyroidism. Like everyone else who has silent lymphocytic thyroiditis, postpartum women go through a hyperthyroid stage, then a hypothyroid stage. During the first phase, their (mild) symptoms may include insomnia, restlessness, anxiety, and poor concentration. The hypothyroid period can bring on fatigue and weight gain. If depression is in the mix, it will most likely appear at this time.

Acute suppurative thyroiditis

There is another rare form of thyroiditis to consider: acute suppurative thyroiditis. It occurs mostly in children and young adults and is caused by a bacterial infection in the thyroid gland. Inflammation takes hold of the thyroid, and pus forms inside. The bacteria can arise from any part of the body, including the throat. Like many other bacterial infections, this one can cause the thyroid to hurt and bring on a high fever. At times the illness may feel like the flu. Pain in the thyroid gland is the main tipoff that the infection may not be the result of more common thyroid maladies. The cure for acute suppurative thyroiditis is antibiotics and surgery to drain the pus.

Riedel's thyroiditis

This is a rare form of thyroiditis in which the thyroid-gland tissue gradually hardens into dense fibers similar to those of scar tissue. As the thyroid tissue is taken over by these tissues, the gland loses its ability to make thyroid hormone and hypothyroidism sets in. The only recourse is surgery (see page, 58–62) to remove the fibers.

Lymphocytic thyroiditis

This long-term thyroiditis is also known as Hashimoto's disease (see page 38).

Thyroid lumps
doctors call them nodules

A thyroid **nodule** is a medical word for a lump of tissue that forms on or near the thyroid gland. Such lumps are common, usually painless, and rarely malignant (cancerous). Each year about a quarter of a million people are found to have thyroid nodules, and millions more may have nodules that go unnoticed because the nodules behave themselves. In some cases, a benign nodule will start to overproduce thyroid hormone and cause hyperthyroidism. When this happens, the nodule is then referred to as a **toxic nodule**.

Who finds these nodules? Well, you do, if you are alert enough to notice a lump on the neck (see page 23 to learn how to do a neck check). Other nodules are discovered by doctors. Some nodules may have been just sitting there for years, neither growing nor shrinking. Sometimes nodules pop up all of a sudden. Experts don't know what causes most thyroid nodules to form, but they've pinpointed some risk factors. Women are more likely than men to have a thyroid nodule. But men are more likely to have a cancerous nodule. Having a family history of thyroid problems increases your risk of developing nodules, and so do any preexisting thyroid disorders. Previous treatment of the head or neck with radiation—for example, to treat facial acne—can also increase your chances. The risk of cancer in a thyroid nodule is about 5 percent.

Benign nodules come in different types. Those that contain fluid are called **cysts**. A cyst can be diagnosed by ultrasound. To find out if a nodule contains fluid, doctors conduct a needle biopsy (see pages 68–69). If the nodule does turn out to be a cyst, the fluid can be drawn out and the nodule will collapse. This procedure is fast, safe, and accurate, with very little discomfort associated.

Thyroid lumps that consist of a number of benign, inactive glandular cells are called **adenomas**. These nodules are usually painless, small, and unnoticeable. Over time they may actually shrink a bit. They have no effect on the thyroid or any of its functions. Thyroid blood tests come out normal.

A benign nodule that can dramatically affect thyroid hormone activity is known as a **toxic adenoma.** It's a noncancerous but abnormal growth or lump that first imitates the functions of the thyroid gland and then takes over those functions. Just like a healthy thyroid, a toxic adenoma produces thyroid hormone. The problem is that eventually both the thyroid gland and the toxic adenoma pump out hormones, flooding the bloodstream and soon causing hyperthyroidism. Thyroid stimulating hormone (TSH) has no control over this excess production. If there are several toxic adenomas, the condition is called toxic multinodular goiter, meaning several nodules on an enlarged thyroid.

A **multinodular goiter** is a growth that contains many nodules (lumps). Over time, it's not uncommon for these lumps to affect the thyroid. The result is either hypo- or hyperthyroidism.

Experts point out that even though most nodules are benign, nodules still need to be checked out by a physician. Until they are examined and tested, you cannot be sure that they are harmless (and you don't want to take any chances).

Types of Thyroid Nodules

Name	Benign?	Affects the thyroid?
Cyst	Usually	No
Adenoma	Yes	No
Toxic adenoma	Yes	Yes
Multinodular goiter	Usually	Yes

Helpful resources

The Thyroid Sourcebook
by M. Sara Rosenthal

Thyroid Disease: The Facts
by R.I.S. Bayliss and
W.M.G. Tunbridge

**Thyroid Foundation of
America, Inc.**
Tel: 800 832-8321
Fax: 617 534-1515
www.allthyroid.org

Foundation of Thyroid Patients
Tel: 432 694-9966
www.thyroidfoundation.org

*Merck Manual of Medical
Information*
www.merck.com

Gland Central
(Internet source of thyroid
information)
www.glandcentral.com

Treatments for Thyroid Disorders

What can be done?
choose from a range of treatments

Your doctor has several options for treating thyroid disorders. The choice of treatment depends on several factors: the type of disorder and the severity of your symptoms, your age, your overall health, and your allergies to medication. As with the various thyroid disorders, thyroid treatments fall into several different categories: treatments that redress your hormonal imbalances and treatments that fix structural problems, such as thyroid growths. Often treatment solves both these problems at the same time.

There are three distinct types of treatments:

1. Radioactive iodine treatment

This treatment calls for radiation to purposefully damage an out-of-control thyroid. This can be due to Graves' disease or an invasive thyroid growth. Large doses are used to treat many cases of thyroid cancer.

2. Medicine (either thyroid hormone replacement or thyroid suppression medication)

These prescription medicines can help offset the symptoms of too much thyroid hormone or supplement insufficient thyroid hormone. If you need to boost your supply of thyroid hormone, you will be prescribed either synthetic or natural thyroid hormones. If your thyroid needs to be brought under control, you may be prescribed antithyroid medicine, which will stop the production of excessive thyroid hormone.

3. Surgery

Often the only way to handle large thyroid nodules is to remove them surgically. The same obviously goes for any cancerous thyroid tissue. Surgery is used to remove benign nodules that are unsightly or restricting breathing by constricting the windpipe. Surgery can also be used for people with Graves' disease who do not want radioactive iodine or to be on long-term antithyroid medication.

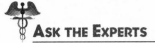

Could my thyroid problem be the result of another underlying condition?

There are a number of serious illnesses that can decrease the levels of thyroid hormones in your blood, namely diabetes and certain liver diseases. However, these diseases do not affect the function of your thyroid. At the most, they can skew thyroid function tests. In fact, your thyroid hormone levels will often dip down after a cold or short-term illness, but will return to normal in a few weeks. If you are having a thyroid test, be sure to tell your doctor if you have recently recovered from a cold or flu.

My doctor told me there is a chance my hyperthyroidism can develop into hypothyroidism. Is this right?

Yes. Any treatment that impairs the thyroid, such as radioactive iodine, surgery, or antithyroid medication can create hypothyroidism. That's because sometimes the only way to stop a thyroid that is in overdrive is, essentially, to turn it off completely. This is a viable option because hypothyroidism is treatable by taking daily doses of thyroid hormone.

Treatments—not a cure

For most thyroid disorders, there is no known cure, there is only treatment to mitigate the symptoms. That can be a hard fact to swallow. For many people the fact that their thyroid disorder is "incurable" is demoralizing. But try to look at the glass as half full. A hundred years ago, a diagnosis of Hashimoto's or Graves' disease would have been a death sentence. That is no longer the case. While treatment does not cure, it does stop the problem in its tracks. For most people, all they need is a pill a day and they are just fine.

Radioactive iodine treatment
an ingenious solution

Radioactive iodine is the treatment of choice for most people with hyper-thyroidism. It is an ingenious treatment because it targets only your thyroid cells. This is because your thyroid is the only part of your body that uses iodine. The thyroid converts iodine from foods that we ingest into thyroid hormones. In hyperthyroidism, the thyroid has gone into overdrive, so there are now too many thyroid cells that are grabbing onto too much iodine and therefore producing too much thyroid hormone. The most effective way to stop this overproduction is to kill off some of the excess thyroid cells. One way to do that is to ingest radioactive iodine so when thyroid cells begin to grab the radioactive iodine, they are put out of commission.

In this treatment people take the radioactive iodine medicine in a pill or in a drink of water. Either way, the iodine is tasteless. The thyroid always soaks up iodine to manufacture hormones, so it quickly takes up the radioactive iodine, which easily seeps into the thyroid cells. The radioactivi-ty in the iodine destroys the cells, the thyroid shrinks, and hormone pro-duction decreases dramatically. Over the next few days the radioactive iodine leaves your system, mostly through your urine.

The challenge your doctor faces is to eradicate just enough thyroid cells to get your hormone levels back to normal without destroying so many cells that hypothyroidism sets in. Most people need only one treatment to signif-icantly lower hormone levels and halt the hyperthyroidism. Sometimes, though, a second treatment is necessary.

In most people the hyperthyroidism disappears in three to six months. In fact, about 90 percent of those who take this treatment gain permanent control over their hyperthyroidism. On the downside, a large majority of people will also develop hypothyroidism, a condition that can be controlled with daily doses of synthetic thyroid hormones (see pages 54–55).

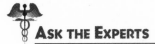

ASK THE EXPERTS

Fiction. The amount of radiation used to treat hyperthyroidism is so tiny that it does not pose a risk of any kind of cancer.

It is not advisable for pregnant women to undergo this treatment. People who are allergic to iodine or shellfish (which contains iodine) should not use this treatment.

This is a new experimental technique that is being developed to treat a number of disorders, one of which is hyperthyroidism. This technique uses a laser beam to destroy the thyroid arteries, thereby disabling the thyroid. As reported in the *Journal of Clinical Endocrinological Metabolism* in 2002, arterial embolization has been shown to be an excellent alternative for people who cannot tolerate surgery, medication, or RAI, such as the elderly.

Medication

medicine to adjust hormonal imbalances

The twenty-first century is full of many medical wonders, none more spectacular than the ability of science to mimic the powers of the body's natural chemicals, the hormones. This is good news because ultimately most people with serious thyroid disorders need help to counter their hormonal imbalances. They either have an abundance of thyroid hormone and need medicine to stop that—called antithyroid medication—or they need to take thyroid hormones to supplement their insufficient thyroid hormone.

Medication to treat thyroid disorders can affect your thyroid and its operations through several different biochemical actions: (1) altering the way thyroid hormone is transported through your system, (2) interfering with the metabolic processing of thyroid hormone, (3) changing how your body regulates hormone production, or (4) blocking the action of hormones on tissues.

The Elegance of Iodine

One key way hypothyroid medication works is to harness the power of iodine. To work properly, your thyroid needs something that it can't produce itself: iodine. This element is found in water and in certain foods such as shellfish, milk products, and iodized salt. A normal thyroid will grab just enough iodine from your diet and use it to make thyroid hormones. An underactive thyroid will grow extra cells (inadvertently creating a goiter) to allow it to grab onto more iodine. An overactive thyroid will race through its iodine supply. One solution is to interfere with the thyroid's ability to utilize iodine. That's what most hyperthyroid medicine does.

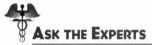

ASK THE EXPERTS

I was told not to take certain medications since I started my thyroid hormone therapy. Why is that?

Any time you take medicine, you need to be on the alert for possible drug interaction with any other medication you need to take. This applies to both prescription and over-the-counter medications. When it comes to thyroid hormonal medicine, there are a number of prescription drug interactions to be wary of (see page 57 for a complete list). Over-the-counter antacids, calcium supplements, iron, and high doses of aspirin can also impede the effects of your thyroid medication. Doctors advise taking them several hours after your thyroid medication.

How can I be sure I don't run into a drug interaction problem?

Make sure your doctor and pharmacist know exactly what medications you are taking, including over-the-counter medicine. If you are taking a number of medications for other conditions, do a brown bag check-up every six months. Simply put all your pills in a brown paper bag and take them to your doctor, who can check them for possible problems. It's a good idea to schedule an appointment with your doctor specifically for this brown-bag examination. It's also a good idea to make a list of all your medications and carry this list with you in case of emergencies.

My doctor prescribed prednisone to treat my thyroiditis. Is that dangerous?

Corticosteroids such as prednisone are used to reduce the swelling of inflamed tissue, making them effective against thyroiditis. Be sure to follow your doctor's dosage instructions; stopping corticosteroids suddenly can cause symptoms to return with a vengeance.

Hyperthyroid medication
antithyroid medicine

When the thyroid goes into overdrive, the only recourse is to neutralize it with radioactive iodine (see page 48) or medicine that cuts back on its over-production of thyroid hormone. (Surgery is also an option; see page 58.) There are two antithyroid drugs. One is the generic propylthiouracil, or **PTU**. It is supplied in 50 mg tablets. The other drug is **methimazole**. It is sold under the brand name Tapazole. It comes in 5 mg and 10 mg tablets. These drugs work by blocking the uptake of iodine into the thyroid cells. Without iodine, the thyroid cannot make thyroid hormone.

About 10 percent of people treated with these drugs experience one or more side effects: allergic reactions (mostly rashes), sore throat, fever, joint pain, loss of taste, and in rare cases a low white blood-cell count, which can leave people vulnerable to infections. Side effects usually disappear when the drugs are withdrawn. Physicians urge patients to call them immediately if, while taking one of these drugs, they develop signs of an infection such as a sore throat or fever, which could signal a low white blood-cell count.

The majority of people treated with these drugs will see their hyperthy-roid symptoms disappear; that is, the symptoms are brought under control. This turnaround can take six weeks to three months. But only a minority of people will actually get permanent relief from the disorder. The vast majori-ty will have to remain on the medication for life in order to remain symp-tom free. In such cases, doctors may also prescribe a small dose of thyroid hormones to normalize your hormone levels. This is called "block and replace." However, few endocrinologists do this anymore, since they can now prescribe such precise amounts of antithyroid medication that normal thyroid hormone production is assured.

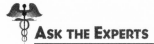

ASK THE EXPERTS

I was just diagnosed with hyperthyroidism. My doctor prescribed something called a beta-blocker. What is that?

Beta-blockers such as metoprolol and propranolol are the other main category of drugs used to treat thyroid symptoms, not the underlying condition. These drugs work to quiet certain parts of the nervous system that have been overstimulated by your thyroid disorder. Doctors prescribe beta-blockers to slow a rapid heartbeat, decrease shakiness, ease anxiety—all of which are hyperthyroid symptoms. Beta-blockers work within hours and can dampen symptoms of anxiety and jitters. If you feel lightheaded or dizzy after taking a beta-blocker, call your doctor.

I've been on my antithyroid medication now for three months and I still feel awful. What can I do?

This is one of the hard parts of having thyroid disease. Not only does it take time for antithyroid medicine to eliminate your symptoms, but it also takes time to hit upon the right dosage. The thyroid influences a myriad of bodily functions. Getting the right amount of thyroid hormone can be a frustrating experience. There is a lot of trial and error. Note: Taking too much can cause anxiety and weight loss as well as lead to osteoporosis and possible atrial fibrillation (irregular heartbeat).

Are there any drugs that adversely interact with hyperthyroidism that I should know about?

When your thyroid is overactive, your whole system is revved up. So the last thing you need is a substance that can speed you up even more. The following can overstimulate your heart: caffeine, tobacco, alcohol, and some combinations of cold medicines with decongestants. Be sure to check the label of any over-the-counter cold medicine before you take it. See pages 56–57 for prescription drug interactions.

Hypothyroid medication

thyroid hormone supplements

In the past, people with thyroid disorders had very little choice of treatment. If they had Hashimoto's disease, they could only watch as they slipped into hypothryoidism. Then, in the nineteenth century, doctors discovered that if their thyroid patients ingested small bits of thyroids from pigs and cows they might indirectly get a helping of the animals' thyroid hormones. And indeed they did. The animal thyroid hormones helped the symptoms and saved thousands of lives.

These animal thyroid hormones are still being prescribed today under such brand names as Armour Thyroid and Thyroid Strong. The advantage of these natural hormones is that they contain both T_3 and T_4 hormones. The disadvantage is that it is difficult to standardize the actual content of these natural drugs. For this reason, scientists came up with synthetic hormones. They created hormones for each specific hormone. The main brand name for T_4 is Synthroid; for T_3 it's Cytomel. If you need a combination of T_4 and T_3 you may be prescribed Thyrolar.

The need for T_3 is still under debate. Some doctors think that T_4 alone can treat hypothyroidism; others find that T_3 needs to be added to the therapy, especially for patients who have been "normalized" on synthetic T_4 replacement therapy but still suffer from confusion, depression, lethargy, and impaired mental functioning. After receiving T_3 replacement, the majority of patients feel like themselves again. For more on the T_3 debate see pages 202–203.

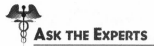

ASK THE EXPERTS

How do doctors know how much thyroid hormone to prescribe?

Doctors try to estimate the right dose by considering how much is needed to normalize TSH levels, the person's age, and any other diseases that may be present. They start out prescribing a six-week round of thyroid therapy and then test your TSH levels to see if they have normalized. They keep increasing the dose in 30-day cycles until your TSH is stable.

I am pregnant and was just diagnosed with hypothyroidism. Is there a connection?

Pregnancy increases the levels of estrogen in the body. Because estrogen can bind T_4 to proteins in the blood, it lowers the amount of thyroid hormone in the body. The result is hypothyroidism. To counteract that, doctors usually prescribe thyroid medicine. The dose is scaled back after delivery.

How to take your hormone pills

◆ Take your thyroid hormone pill on an empty stomach. If you can, take your thyroid hormone two hours before having a meal or taking vitamins.

◆ Take your hormone pill separately from any other medications you might have. Keep your thyroid pills in a place that will help you remember to take them, such as next to your toothbrush.

◆ If you forget to take your thyroid pill, skip it and take your next regular dose at the regular time.

◆ Take your medicine at the same time every day.

Drug interactions
what to look out for

Some prescription and over-the-counter medications don't mix well with synthetic thyroid hormone. They can blunt the effects of your thyroid hormone or increase it. Conversely, thyroid medication can affect various prescription drugs, causing them to become too effective or ineffective. Unfortunately, the list of offending drugs is long. For the most part these drugs increase or reduce the effectiveness of your synthetic hormone by either delaying or preventing absorption. What can you do to avoid this problem? Experts recommend taking these at different times than your dose of synthetic hormone. Always tell your doctor if you are taking any other medications.

Medications that can speed up the processing of synthetic hormone in the liver, sometimes causing hypothyroidism, include carbamazepine, phenobarbital, and rifampin.

Medications that can be rendered ineffective by synthetic thyroid hormone include oral anticoagulants, such as warfarin, that help "thin" the blood to prevent strokes and heart attacks. When they're taken with synthetic hormone, however, their clot-busting power may be reduced. Physicians recommend close monitoring of people who take these two types of medications together.

Drugs that can increase the side effects of both the hormone and the prescribed drugs include three types of antidepressants—tricyclics, tetracyclics, and selective serotonin reuptake inhibitors (SSRIs). These effects may include irregular heartbeat and stimulation of the central nervous system.

Adding thyroid hormone to certain antidiabetic or insulin therapy may increase the body's requirement for these diabetes drugs. Doctors recommend careful monitoring of the following drugs when combined with synthetic thyroid: meglitinides, sulfonylureas, and insulin.

Drugs that can cause or aggravate hypothyroidism

Trade Name	Brand Names	Treatment For
Acetazolamide	Ak-Zol, Diamox, Daranide	convulsions, glaucoma
Aluminum Hydroxide	Maalox, Mylanta, Amphogel	ulcers
Aminoglutethimide	Cytadren	tumors
Amiodarone	Cordarone, Pacerone	irregular heart rhythms
Aspirin	Bayer, Anacin, Buffrin	inflammation, blood clots
Carbamazepine	Atretol, Carbatrol, Epitol	convulsions, seizures
Cholestyramine	Questran	high cholesterol levels
Colestipol	Colestid	high cholesterol, blood fats
Diphenylhydantoin	Dilantin, Cerebyx	convulsions, seizures
Estrogen	Premarin, Estinyl, Estrace	menopause, birth control
Glucocorticoid	Aristocort, Hydrocortone, Prednisone	inflammation, asthma, arthritis
Lithium	Lithane, Lithobid, Eskalith	bipolar disorders
Methimazole	Tapazole	hyperthyroidism
Propranolol	Cartrol, Inderal, Levatol	high blood pressure, angina

Thyroid surgery
another option

Thyroid surgery is used to remove thyroid growths. Sometimes these growths (nodules or goiters) are part of an underlying thyroid problem that is causing you to experience hypo- or hyperthyroid symptoms. But often they appear for no apparent reason. Surgery is an option if:

◆ You are allergic to iodine or other thyroid medication.

◆ Your airway is blocked or compressed.

◆ You have a benign nodule that's producing too much thyroid hormone (and causing hyperthyroidism) or is pressing against your airway or voice box.

◆ You have a massive goiter that can't be eliminated any other way.

◆ You have, or are suspected of having, thyroid cancer (see pages 65–80). In this case, only surgery holds out the possibility of eradicating all cancerous tumors.

Thyroid surgery is a fairly low-risk procedure. There is a slight chance that the voice box may be damaged, causing problems with normal speech. The parathyroid gland, a small organ near the thyroid, can also be injured, disrupting control of calcium levels in the blood. Because thyroid surgery involves removing thyroid tissue there is always a chance that it will result in hypothyroidism, which is usually corrected with life-long, daily doses of thyroid hormone (see page 54).

There are three types of thyroid surgery: a partial lobectomy, a full lobectomy, and a thyroidectomy.

Partial lobectomy A lobectomy is the surgical removal of one lobe of the thyroid gland, so a partial lobectomy is the removal of part of one lobe. The usual purpose of this rarely performed procedure is to remove a single nodule. This nodule can be unsightly or cancerous or causing hyperthyroid symptoms.

Full lobectomy In this procedure one whole thyroid lobe is removed. Doctors often prefer to remove the entire lobe even though they are only after a single nodule on a lobe. Very often the final decision on how much thyroid gland and other tissue to remove is made during surgery. While operating, the surgeon may take a sample of tissue, send it to the lab for quick examination, and decide the extent of the surgery after checking the lab report.

Thyroidectomy Surgeons often disagree on how much tissue should be removed if cancerous nodules are found. Some prefer to perform just a full lobectomy only if the cancerous tumors (see page 78) are small and not very aggressive. If there's evidence from a biopsy suggesting malignancy, some surgeons opt to remove almost all of the thyroid gland (a procedure called a subtotal thyroidectomy). Others will go further still and perform a total thyroidectomy, removing all thyroid tissue. A total thyroidectomy may include nearby lymph nodes, an operation designed to prevent metastases, the spread of cancer.

Cutting-Edge Treatments

Another advance involves injecting ethanol, or pure alcohol, directly into "hot nodules" (ones that produce hyperthyroidism) instead of ablating (destroying) them with radioactive iodine treatments (RAI) or removing them surgically. The ethanol kills the blood supply to the thyroid. This technique has been shown to be superior to RAI, which often destroys the entire thyroid gland, resulting in hypothyroidism in 40% of patients. For now, this procedure is available only in Italy.

Thyroid operations
what goes on during an operation

What actually happens during thyroid surgery? During the operation the surgeon carefully makes an incision across the neck where the thyroid is, trying to follow a skin fold to minimize scarring. The incision is three to five inches long, and the entire operation is performed through this small opening. It is extremely rare for an infection or other problem to accompany this incision. The surgeon gets a pretty good view of the thyroid gland, checking for nodules and any signs that cancer has spread to the lymph nodes. Based on this examination, she will decide how much tissue should be removed and from where.

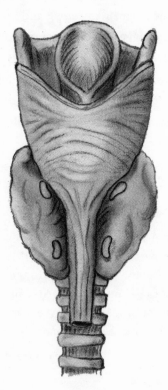

The actual removal of tissue is tricky and requires an experienced hand. The thyroid is a small gland. Moreover, there are blood vessels running the length of the throat and passing through the thyroid. There are several parathyroid glands (shown here in blue) in the area as well as nerves leading to the voice box. The surgeon tries to eliminate thyroid tissue without harming these structures. Damage to the parathyroid glands could cause a drop in blood calcium levels, and an injury to the voice box could result in temporary or permanent hoarseness.

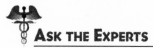

ASK THE EXPERTS

Will I have stitches after thyroid surgery?

Yes, but probably only one. Usually a single stitch is all that's needed to secure the incision. Before you leave the hospital, the stitch is removed and a clear protective bandage is applied to the wound. With the incision protected, you can shower without worrying that you will damage it.

Will I have a scar after thyroid surgery?

Yes, but it will fade over the next few months, probably becoming barely noticeable. Good surgeons know several techniques for reducing the likelihood of a noticeable scar, including making the smallest possible cut across the skin and avoiding inflammation and infection in the incision. If you have a concern about scarring, discuss it with your surgeon.

How can I find a good surgeon to perform this surgery?

There are several ways. Ask your family physician for a referral, or contact thyroid support organizations to see if they offer a list of thyroid experts categorized by geographical area. Such organizations include the American Thyroid Association (**www.thyroid.org**) and the American Association of Endocrine Surgeons (**www.endocrinesurgeons.org**). In the end the only criterion that matters is how much experience a doctor has in thyroid surgery. Good candidates should have performed thyroid surgery hundreds of times and currently perform thyroid operations several times a week or month.

How do doctors check to see whether the surgery did what it was supposed to do?

After surgery for thyroid cancer, they will run a standard radioactive iodine scan of the thyroid to check whether there is any sign of cancer. They may also do blood tests to measure thyroid function.

Why is surgery used to treat hyperthyroidism?

Hyperthyroidism is the result of too much thyroid hormone in your bloodstream. So anything that prevents the thyroid from making so much hormone will help alleviate the overactive thyroid. Thyroidectomy is one way to quickly reduce or eliminate the gland's output of hormone. The decision to have the thyroidectomy will depend on how big the goiter is, the failure of other treatments (e.g., radioactive iodine), whether the goiter is pressing too hard against structures in the throat, whether thyroid eye disease is a major concern, and other factors.

Why do some people require a second thyroid operation?

Occasionally some surgeons will recommend a second operation after reexamining the patient's thyroid. The reexamination may reveal that a malignancy has returned, and removing the last remnant of the thyroid gland may be the best way to deal with it. This kind of recurrence of cancer suggests to many surgeons that the first operation should have been more extensive. At other times a second operation may be necessary to deal with a noncancerous thyroid problem, such as a goiter or recurring hyperthyroidism.

How many thyroid surgeries should a doctor perform before he or she is considered "experienced?"

The New York Thyroid Center has issued guidelines for answering this question. They suggest that a surgeon's experience should be judged by the number of thyroid or parathyroid operations performed. If a surgeon has performed less than 200, he or she is "inexperienced." If 200 to 500, "intermediate"; over 500, "experienced"; and over 1,000, "expert."

I was just diagnosed with Hashimoto's disease and my doctor immediately put me on synthetic hormone replacement therapy. Is that the right thing to do?

The rationale is that hormone treatment can prevent the inevitable hypothyroidism and possible goiters from ever arising. The hormone replacement, though, usually must be taken daily for life.

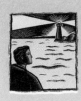

FIRST PERSON INSIGHTS

I've got the beep!

My doctor wanted to do a radioactive iodine test on my thyroid. She said it was the best way to check on the shape, position, and functioning of my thyroid. It sounded so high-tech and scary, but it was a pretty easy test. The radiologist technician checked me for any allergic reaction to iodine. I was negative for that. He told me to avoid any thyroid medication or drugs that contained iodine for two weeks before the test. I went to the lab on the appointed day and was given a pill to swallow and told to report back the next day. I was asked to lie down, and the technician placed a small radioactive detector over my neck. I could hear the beeps going off. Basically, it's a Geiger counter. The technician recorded the number of beeps as I watched them bounce on the computer screen. It was a little disconcerting, but painless. I felt like I was in a science-fiction movie. After 30 minutes, the test was over and I could get up and go home. Phew. The test revealed that I had Graves' disease and I started treatment.

—Anne S., Minneapolis, MN

Helpful resources

Mosby's Diagnostic and Laboratory Test Reference
by Kathleen Pagana and
Timothy Pagana

The Thyroid Sourcebook
by M. Sara Rosenthal

Thyroid Disease, The Facts
by R.I.S. Bayliss and
W.M.G. Tunbridge

Thyroid Foundation of America, Inc.
Tel: 800 832-8321
Fax: 617 534-1515
www.allthyroid.org

American Foundation of Thyroid Patients
Tel: 432 694-9966
www.thyroidfoundation.org

Merck Manual of Medical Information
www.merck.com

Gland Central
(Internet source of thyroid information)
glandcentral.com

Thyroid Cancer

Examining the thyroid
what is that lump?

Usually the first clue that you have a thyroid problem is a lump in the neck area, either on the thyroid or nearby. Sometimes you are the one to first detect the lump; sometimes your doctor is. Such lumps often turn out to be benign nodules, goiters, or a swelling due to thyroid infection or inflammation. But in 5 percent of cases they are cancerous. The good news is that thyroid cancer is very treatable, with a very high cure rate.

Once a lump is detected, your doctor's first step will be to do a physical exam of the neck, thyroid, windpipe, and lymph glands. She may decide to reexamine the lump in a few weeks. Frequently, by then the lump will have grown smaller or disappeared, a sign that it is benign. If your doctor thinks the lump is suspicious (either before or after a wait-and-see period), she may want to do further testing. There are several clues that might make your doctor suspicious enough to investigate the lump further:

◆ History of thyroid trouble in you or your family.

◆ Radiation exposure when you were a child (not including radioactive iodine treatments or tests).

◆ The presence of a single nodule rather than several, especially if the nodule grows quickly.

◆ A painless, hard lump on your thyroid or neck.

◆ Male patient (because nodules are more likely to be cancerous in men than in women).

◆ A nodule that's getting bigger and bigger, despite treatment with thyroid hormone.

◆ Young patient (because nodules are more likely to be cancerous in children).

Don't ignore bumps or lumps

I was a healthy 44-year-old woman when one day I happened to discover a lump on my thyroid. I pressed on it, but it didn't hurt, so I just ignored it. I had had the flu a few weeks back and figured this lump was probably from that. Still, it bothered me. I noticed that when I stood in front of the mirror and swallowed, the lump would move up and down. After a few weeks, I saw that it wasn't going away. I figured no lumps were good lumps so I made an appointment with my doctor. I was pretty shocked to learn that the lump was actually a nodule on my thyroid gland. I was even more concerned to learn that it had to be checked out because there was a chance that it was cancerous.

My doctor scheduled me to have a fine-needle biopsy. When the biopsy report came back from the lab, he told me the news: "It's good that we did the biopsy," he said, "because the lump is malignant."

I was stunned. *Cancer* is such a scary word. How could this happen to me? I think I even teared up. My doctor explained that the treatment of choice for my kind of cancer is surgery. And even though my nodule was small, he preferred to remove the entire lobe, just in case. He scheduled me for surgery the next week, and I was home the same day of the surgery. I had no real symptoms except a raspy voice for a few days. I then had to get thyroid blood tests every month or two for a year and then every six months. It's been four years, and I am fine.

—Margaret C., Bedford, NY

Diagnostic tests
how they work

Your doctor's next step will be to run tests for signs of cancer. To do this, he may refer you to an endocrinologist or a head and neck surgeon (see pages 114–115). An endocrinologist knows a lot about thyroid disorders; a head and neck surgeon knows a lot about different types of neck lumps.

The definitive test is a biopsy (extracting a sample of tissue to check it for cancer). Ultimately, doing a biopsy is the only way to be sure that cancer is present. The usual biopsy method is the fine-needle aspiration. This involves inserting a thin needle into a thyroid nodule to take some cells for analysis. The cell sample is put under a microscope and checked to see if the cells are malignant or likely to become malignant. In cases in which a fine-needle aspiration cannot be done, a surgical biopsy is performed. The whole nodule is removed and then examined for cancer cells.

Though a biopsy can give a definitive answer about the existence of cancer, doctors often use other tests along with it. Sometimes these tests are done before a biopsy is performed as a way to check for benign nodules, to ascertain how many nodules are present, to rule out benign conditions such as hyper- or hypothyroidism, or to provide additional information about a suspicious nodule. These tests include:

- ◆ **Blood tests** (see page 18) to check the levels of thyroid-stimulating hormone (TSH).

- ◆ **Thyroid scans** (see page 20) to check how much radioactive iodine a lump absorbs. Benign nodules usually absorb a lot of iodine because they are functioning as the rest of the thyroid does, taking in iodine. On the scan picture, such nodules, called "hot" nodules, will be darker than surrounding tissue. Cancerous nodules are almost always "cold" nodules, indicating that they are not absorbing iodine. However, since so few nodules are hot and not all cold nodules are cancerous, doctors usually do an ultrasound and a biopsy to be sure.

◆ **Ultrasound** to get a closer look at the nodules. An ultrasound bounces sound waves off the thyroid to create a picture of the gland's interior. An ultrasound picture (called a sonogram) can reveal the number of nodules as well as their size and whether they are filled with fluid and are therefore cysts.

◆ **Biopsy** to check for cancer status. Doctors will do a biopsy to determine whether there are any cancerous cells.

◆ **Staging** to discover if the cancer has spread to the lymph nodes or other parts of the neck. To do accurate staging, doctors use several kinds of test, including ultrasound, magnetic resonance imaging (MRI), and computerized axial tomography (CT, or CAT scan). To find out if the cancer has extended to distant parts of the body, they look at the whole body using radioactive iodine scanning.

Questions to Ask Your Doctor about Biopsies

Why am I having this biopsy?

What kind of biopsy will I have?

Who will perform the biopsy? Where? How long will it take?

Will it hurt?

Will the biopsy leave a scar?

When will I know the biopsy results?

Will the person doing the biopsy be the same person who does any subsequent surgery?

When it's thyroid cancer
risk factors

Thyroid cancer is the most curable type of cancer. In fact, well over 90 percent of thyroid cancer cases are curable. This track record is understandable once you know that cancer of the thyroid, compared to other cancers, is not very aggressive. Generally, thyroid cancer grows slowly (so slowly that it could take a decade or two to even begin to reach other organs). This sluggishness gives doctors plenty of time to detect it, which is why it is almost always diagnosed in its earliest stages. If it's allowed to grow unchecked for a long time, then it can be lethal. But nowadays this is rare. And if treatment is required, it typically can be done with minimal pain and disability.

Though the chances of your having thyroid cancer are low, there are factors that can increase your risk.

At the top of the list is **radiation**. Decades ago, doctors used X-rays to treat children with various ailments related to the head and neck, such as acne and enlarged tonsils. Years later an unusually large proportion of these people developed thyroid cancer. So doctors abandoned the use of X-ray treatments for benign conditions. (Today's X-rays are for diagnostic purposes, involve very low doses of X-rays, and come with minimal risks.) Adults who had X-ray treatments as a child, though, are now at a higher risk of developing thyroid cancer.

Family history can also affect your chances of getting thyroid cancer. A particular kind of thyroid malignancy, called medullary thyroid cancer, can sometimes run in families. Using a blood test, your doctor can tell if you have the genetic abnormality that leads to this kind of cancer. If someone has medullary thyroid cancer, then his or her close relatives should be screened through genetic testing.

A **low-iodine** diet can also increase your risk of getting thyroid cancer. Iodine deficiency is rare in the United States because iodine is added to table salt. Other areas of the world are not so lucky. In parts of China, Africa, Russia, and other countries, millions of people have iodine deficiency, which is a major cause of mental retardation.

There are several other factors that raise the risk of thyroid cancer. The first is age—the majority of people with thyroid cancer are over 40 years old. Race is another factor; thyroid cancer is more likely to occur in Caucasians than in African Americans. Finally, gender plays a role. Women in the United States are up to three times more likely to have thyroid cancer than men. But that's because nodules are so much more common in women. That said, a nodule in a man is more likely to be cancerous than a nodule in a woman.

But what does having one or more of these risk factors really mean? It does not mean that you are sure to develop thyroid cancer. Most people with risk factors don't get cancer of the thyroid, and some people who develop thyroid cancer have no risk factors at all. That's why testing is so key.

Being Told You Have Cancer

Getting a diagnosis of any kind of cancer is scary. The very word *cancer* connotes such dire images of pain and suffering in some people that they are afraid to even use the word in everyday conversation. Should you be told that you have thyroid cancer, don't be frightened. Thyroid cancer is extremely curable. And don't give way to any feelings of guilt for somehow causing the cancer or doing something to trigger it. Medical disorders happen. Short of having a family history of thyroid cancer, there is no real explanation for why you, and not someone else, got thyroid cancer.

Four kinds of thyroid cancer
what are they?

Thyroid cancer is not one disease but many. In fact, there are four distinct types of thyroid cancer: papillary, follicular, medullary, and anaplastic. Each of these types of cancer differs in what causes it, how it grows, how it's diagnosed, how it's treated, and how easy or difficult it is to eradicate. The one thing they share is that they all begin with wayward cells that combine to form lumps of tissue, or malignant tumors. Treatment is fairly straightforward. The first step is usually partial or complete removal of the thyroid (see pages 58–63), followed by either doses of thyroid hormone or radioactive iodine treatment. Often the therapy finishes with daily doses of synthetic thyroid hormone. Why do you need thyroid medication? Because thyroid-hormone supplements can suppress the growth of new tumors, and with the removal of the thyroid you need hormone replacement.

Papillary thyroid cancer is the most prevalent type of thyroid cancer, accounting for 60 to 70 percent of thyroid malignancies. *Papillary* refers to a papilla, a nipplelike protrusion, which describes the appearance of tiny papillary growths. This kind of thyroid cancer occurs mostly in women and shows up predominantly in adults aged 30 to 50. In this group it grows slowly and is highly curable. When it occurs in older adults, it grows and spreads faster than it does in younger people. Papillary cancer is the type most likely to result from exposure to radiation.

Cancer cells in one part of the body can sometimes spread to other sites, a process called metastasis. Papillary thyroid cancer cells can metastasize to the lymph glands in the neck. But even when they do, the usual good prognosis for patients does not change. In a very small percentage of people with this kind of cancer, cancer cells spread beyond the lymph glands to other parts of the body. Even in this case the cancer can usually be effectively treated with radioactive iodine.

Follicular thyroid cancer gets its name from the tiny sphere-shaped structures called follicles that make up a normal thyroid gland. Follicular thyroid cancer accounts for 25 percent of all cases of thyroid cancer, affecting women much more than men and occurring more frequently over the age of 50 than under.

This thyroid cancer is generally more aggressive than papillary cancer, meaning that it can spread more easily from the thyroid to other parts of the body. This aggressive course happens in about two-thirds of people with the cancer. In the other third, the cancer usually does not spread and has a very high cure rate. When follicular thyroid cancer is aggressive, it can invade the bloodstream and scatter to distant tissues, especially the lungs and bones. Treatment for this tougher variety of follicular cancer is also aggressive, usually involving removal of all or part of the thyroid, plus radioactive iodine to kill any remaining cancer cells.

Medullary thyroid cancer is rarer than either papillary or follicular cancer, accounting for only 2 to 8 percent of thyroid malignancies. Most of the time, medullary cancer appears randomly, but it also runs in families and can show up among other gland-type cancers in a condition known as multiple endocrine neoplasia syndrome (MEN). Because of the hereditary nature of the cancer, doctors urge people diagnosed with it to have other members of their family checked. Unlike other thyroid malignancies, medullary cancer occurs in men about as often as in women.

Medullary cancer grows slowly but aggressively, often metastasizing to the lymph nodes as well as the liver, lungs, and bones. If it is detected before spreading, the chances of treating it successfully are good. After the cancer begins to spread, treatment is more difficult. In any case, 50 to 70 percent of people with medullary cancer live 10 years or more. The recommended treatment for this malignancy is complete thyroidectomy plus the removal of any tumors in the neck and elsewhere if possible.

Anaplastic thyroid cancer is the rarest of all thyroid malignancies, accounting for just 1 to 2 percent of thyroid cancers and occurring mostly in people over 50. It is also the most dangerous thyroid cancer. Unlike all the other thyroid malignancies, anaplastic cancer spreads quickly and is usually fatal. Both surgery and radioactive iodine therapy have no effect on this cancer. Often by the time this cancer is diagnosed, it has metastasized so thoroughly that surgery becomes irrelevant. Chemotherapy and external radiation therapy likewise have little effect in eradicating the cancer, but they may increase survival time by a few months.

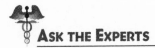

ASK THE EXPERTS

How do people find out that they have thyroid cancer?

Most of the time, either they notice a painless lump on their neck and ask their doctor about it, or their doctor notices it first. Nine times out of ten, the lump is benign. In any case, the doctor will examine the lump and, occasionally, order some tests or refer the case to a specialist. The specialist in treating thyroid problems is known as an endocrinologist, an M.D. who deals with glands. Confirmation that the lump is cancerous typically comes from a biopsy.

Are some malignant thyroid tumors more dangerous than others?

Yes, but doctors try to be more precise about differences in the seriousness of thyroid cancer by talking about stages of thyroid malignancy. A widely used system for doing this categorizes thyroid cancer into one of four possible stages, ranging from Stage 1 (which indicates the presence of a small tumor that has not spread to the lymph nodes) to Stage 4 (which indicates either a very large tumor or one that has spread to both lymph nodes and sites outside the neck).

Can I have more than one type of thyroid cancer at the same time?

Yes. Papillary and follicular cancers often show up together in the same person. The resulting combination is not a less treatable cancer but a more treatable one (that is, more treatable than follicular cancer would be alone).

I told my sister-in-law that I have thyroid cancer. She was supportive, but she wants to tell her mother (my mother-in-law) that I have it. My mother-in-law is elderly and tends to get upset easily. I don't see the need to tell her. What should I do?

Your sister-in-law should not intervene on your behalf, especially if you made it clear that your health information was for her ears only. It could be that your sister-in-law has some unresolved feelings about your health problems. Ask her why she wants to talk to her mother about it. Perhaps she wants to gain some sense of importance by being the messenger of such important news. Or perhaps she merely wishes to add to your support network. Whatever her reason, be firm with her that you do not wish this information to be shared. For more on how to talk to people about your illness, see pages 158–159.

Four stages of cancer
each stage has its own prognosis

If medical tests confirm that you have thyroid cancer, your doctor will not stop there. To treat the tumors effectively, she will also need to know the **stage,** or extent, of your cancer. To determine the stage your cancer is in, your doctor will need to review blood tests, biopsies, as well as MRI body scans. Staging is a way to answer two key questions about your thyroid cancer: Have cancer cells spread from the thyroid to the lymph nodes or other parts of the neck? And have the cancer cells spread to distant sites in the body? Here's the breakdown of stages in the standard staging system:

- ◆ **Stage 1** Cancer cells are confined to the thyroid. (Cancers in Stage 1 are highly treatable and suggest an excellent prognosis.)

- ◆ **Stage 2** Cancer cells are in the thyroid and the lymph nodes. The lymph nodes are enlarged but unattached to surrounding tissue. (Stage 2 cancers are also very treatable and generally lead to a good prognosis.)

- ◆ **Stage 3** Cancer cells extend beyond the thyroid and lymph nodes to other areas of the neck. Cancer cells or lymph nodes are attached to nearby structures. (Stage 3 cancer cells are more difficult to treat, with a recurrence of the cancer in almost one-third of patients. Prognosis is fair.)

- ◆ **Stage 4** Cancer cells have spread beyond the neck to distant sites. (Stage 4 cancers are very difficult to treat. Prognosis is poor.)

Each successive stage indicates a higher recurrence rate and a higher mortality rate. In Stages 1 and 2 (where most thyroid cancers fall), the recurrence and mortality rates are very low. In Stage 1, for example, the recurrence rate is 3 to 5 percent, and the mortality rate is only 1.8 percent.

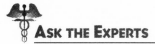

Can my thyroid cancer return after being successfully treated the first time?

Thyroid cancer, like other types of cancer, can recur after being eradicated. The likelihood of this happening is called the recurrence rate, which is the percentage of all successfully treated cancers that reappear. Thyroid cancers have low recurrence rates compared to other kinds of malignancies. Stage 1 thyroid cancer, for instance, has a local recurrence rate of 5.5 percent. *Local recurrence* refers to cancers that reappear in the neck area.

Can people get thyroid cancer from radioactive fallout?

Exposure to radioactive fallout is a risk factor for thyroid cancer, just as exposure to X-ray radiation is. In the 1950s nuclear testing was carried out in Nevada, producing radioactive fallout that migrated into the Midwest. The National Cancer Institute has warned that people (notably children) who lived in the Midwest during the testing are at increased risk for thyroid cancer.

I heard that you can take potassium iodide pills to ward off possible thyroid cancer in the event of a nuclear reactor malfunction. Is that true?

The thyroid is very vulnerable to exposure to radiation. That is why your dentist always covers your neck with a lead apron when taking X-rays of your teeth. In the event of a nuclear disaster, radioactive particles can be released in the air. If that happens, the thyroid is a likely target. One way to protect the thyroid is to take potassium iodide pills. The iodine in the potassium basically blocks the thyroid from absorbing any radioactive iodine. The current wisdom is to take these pills for two weeks when the air quality is compromised. These pills should be taken *only* following a nuclear emergency.

Effective treatment
thyroid cancer is curable

How your doctor treats thyroid cancer depends on several factors—the type of cancer you have, your age, and your general health. One other factor is key: the stage of cancer you have. Its growth rate is rated on a scale from 1 to 4; 1 being slow, 4 being fast.

Stage 1 thyroid cancer is confined to the thyroid only and can consist of a tiny malignant tumor or several larger tumors. This level of cancer is highly treatable and comes with an excellent prognosis. The standard method for dealing with Stage 1 cancer is surgery. Doctors disagree, however, on how extensive the surgery should be. The controversy arises because Stage 1 malignancies have such good prognoses that extensive surgery is not always necessary. The surgical options for Stage 1 cancer include:

◆ Full or partial removal of one lobe of the thyroid, called a lobectomy. (The thyroid is shaped like a butterfly, and each "wing" is a separate lobe. The targeted lobe is the one with the cancerous mass.)

◆ Full removal of one lobe of the thyroid plus partial removal of the other. (This operation takes out a lot of tissue but ensures that little or no damage is done to the windpipe or the parathyroid glands.)

◆ Removal of part or all of the thyroid gland (thyroidectomy) plus radioactive iodine treatment. (The thyroid is removed through an incision in the neck. Partial removal leaves a small bit of the thyroid gland intact to minimize damage to the parathyroid gland and the nerves of the windpipe. Radiation is used to kill any cancer cells that are too small to be detected. Full thyroidectomy risks damage to nearby nerves and glands but improves the probability that all the cancer has been eliminated.)

◆ Full thyroidectomy plus minimal surgery on the neck to look for and remove cancer cells that may have spread to the lymph nodes.

There is much more agreement among doctors about how to treat Stage

2, 3, and 4 cancers than Stage 1 cancers. Doctors generally treat Stage 2 tumors with total (or almost total) thyroidectomy plus removal of malignant or possibly malignant lymph nodes. Surgery is then followed by radioactive iodine treatment.

Doctors take a more aggressive approach with Stage 3 cancer. The usual procedure is to remove the thyroid and take out as much malignant tissue as possible without extensive damage to normal tissue. In Stage 3, cancer invades the thyroid, lymph nodes, and various organs in the neck, including the windpipe, jugular vein, esophagus, and muscles. Doctors remove tumors in these areas; some doctors follow up with external radiation therapy.

In Stage 4, tumors are in the thyroid, lymph nodes, other parts of the neck, and in distant sites such as lungs and bones. Standard treatment is thyroidectomy plus removal of the lymph nodes, neck tumors, and as much of the distant-site cancer as possible. The surgery is followed up with radioactive iodine treatment.

Sometimes after surgery (especially in papillary and follicular cancer) doctors will prescribe synthetic hormone. Thyroid hormone can slow down the growth of any cancer cells that may remain. Often, if patients undergo a total or partial thyroidectomy, they need daily doses of hormone to replace the hormone normally produced by the thyroid.

Questions to Ask Your Doctor Before Surgery

What kind of surgery will I have?

Why do you recommend this type of surgery?

What will be the long-term effects of this surgery? How am I likely to feel a few weeks after the surgery?

What does this type of surgery involve? General anesthesia? Long hospital stay?

Will I have to take thyroid-hormone pills afterward?

Helpful resources

National Cancer Institute
Provides accurate and comprehensive information about many types of cancer, cancer treatments, ongoing scientific studies of thyroid cancer, and more.
http://cancer.gov

The NCI Cancer Information Service
Can answer questions and provide information from the NCI's vast database, PDQ.
Tel: 800-422-6237

The American Thyroid Association
Provides information about thyroid cancer and treatments.
www.thyroid.org

Thyroid Cancer Survivors' Association
Information and support for people with thyroid cancer.
Tel: 877-588-7904
www.thyca.org

Thyroid Foundation of America
Comprehensive information about thyroid disorders.
www.allthyroid.org

EndocrineWeb.com
Answers to common questions about thyroid cancer.
www.endocrineweb.com

The Merck Manual
Authoritative medical information on many diseases, including thyroid cancer.
www.merck.com/pubs/mmanual

Gland Central
www.glandcentral.com

The Johns Hopkins Thyroid Tumor Center
www.thyroid-cancer.net

Using the Internet

Top layman's health sites
the best sites to start with

You have had the tests. And you have been given a diagnosis and perhaps even begun your treatment. If you are like most people, your first instinct is to find out everything there is to know about your thyroid. This is a useful instinct—hold on to it. You don't need to become a thyroid expert your goal is to become an informed, active patient. That's why after seeing their doctor, most people go home, turn on their computer, and start surfing the Internet. You can too. But a word of advice: Don't start by searching through the main search engines, such as AltaVista and Google, since these can overwhelm you with information. Instead, turn to the following sites to become grounded in the basics about the thyroid. Here are three good starting points that are a little more specific.

HealthScout

www.healthscout.com

Type of site: General consumer health site

The HealthScout Network provides health-encyclopedia information and focused news reports for big Web sites like Yahoo, USA Today, and NBCi. You can see at a glance that it's supported by advertising, but that does not get in the way of the content.

Your first port of call should be the HealthScout's encyclopedia. The quickest way to get to the right entry is to enter a keyword or two in the search box on HealthScout's home page. What you will get is a listing of articles and their dates, as well as a percentage figure at the end that tells you how relevant the article is to your keywords. If the figure is 100 percent, it's definitely worth taking a look.

EndocrineWeb

www.endocrineweb.com

Type of site: Disease-specific consumer health site

You can tell by the name that EndocrineWeb is going to get a little more technical. Your body's endocrine system includes all your glands, and EndocrineWeb covers them all. But at the top of the list is the thyroid. Click on the Thyroid link and you will be ready for your course on the thyroid gland. EndocrineWeb's pages are nicely illustrated and read like an intelligent magazine article rather than a crusty academic tome. The articles are just long enough and just technical enough to help you "get" the whole thing.

About.com's Thyroid Disease site

http://thyroid.about.com

Type of site: Disease-specific patient-advocate site

Despite being horribly overburdened with advertising, About.com is a solid resource for information from someone who knows. Mary Shomon, the Web master and editor of the site, has turned her struggle with Hashimoto's thyroiditis into a thoughtful site that presents clear writing and compassion that's often missing from more technical sites. Ms. Shomon's site provides links to other Web sites, but it's her own articles that bring the subject to life—don't miss her "20 Secrets of Successful Thyroid Patients" and "10 Thyroid Mistakes Your Doctor May Be Making."

Getting online

If you don't have Internet access at home, you are not out of luck. Many public libraries have Internet-access stations that you can use for half an hour or more at a stretch—as long as you have a library card.

Top medical-research sites
go to these for clinical information

Once you have a basic grounding in your thyroid condition, you'll be ready to sink your teeth into something more substantial. Again, avoid doing a general search; go instead to the established medical sites. There are two basic types of sites: ones that are maintained by a specific medical school or clinic and the big medical search engines that are supported by the U.S. government.

Medical institutions

Universities and clinics often provide outreach sites for health issues—it makes their medical school or clinic all the more prestigious. And they supply up-to-date information: Academic resources are rigorously checked for accuracy. Here are some of the bigger medical sites run by institutions.

InteliHealth
http://www.intelihealth.com
Johns Hopkins University's excellent and easy-to-understand collection of journal databases, a medical dictionary, and expert Q&As.

Martindale's Health Science Guide
http://www-sci.lib.uci.edu/HSG/HSGuide.html
Extensive database of health-related information, news, and references.

Mayo Clinic
www.mayoclinic.com
The respected clinic's Web site does a great job of making health and medicine issues easy to understand.

National Institutes of Health's Medline
http://www.medlineplus.gov
The prime source of clinical and patient-oriented information. Sometimes tough, but deep and useful.

Medical search engines

Search engines embedded in a reliable medical site are the quickest way to get good information from that site and sometimes other sites that are affiliated with it. The pool you are searching is the smallest, but because of that you will be getting the most relevant results. Here are some examples of medical search engines:

Healthfinder
http://www.healthfinder.gov/
A publication of the U.S. government's National Institutes of Health, Healthfinder's search engine finds pages from prescreened, authoritative sites. The content often doesn't go deep, but it's written in an accessible way.

Medline
http://www.medlineplus.gov
Another site provided by the National Institutes of Health, Medline offers a great deal of clinical information. Enter your search terms here and you will get results with deep research from an encyclopedic government-run source.

Smart searching

Use the phrase that pays. Enter Graves' disease in a search box and your results could be cluttered with reports of any illness the actor Peter Graves or the author Robert Graves ever suffered. Put quote marks around phrases (as in "Graves' disease") and most search engines will exclude results that include isolated uses of each of the words.

Nonprofit research sites
check out the advocacy groups

Nonprofit institutions and societies dedicated to the study, cure, or relief of a particular ailment are another good source of reliable information online. They're not all patient oriented, and they're sometimes contradictory (because professionals love to argue about details), but they can provide very helpful information. Their Web site names tell you exactly what they are about.

American Foundation of Thyroid Patients
www.thyroidfoundation.org

A national, nonprofit organization for the awareness, education, and support of thyroid patients, their family members, health care providers, and other interested parties. Offers support/interest groups forming around America, low-cost public thyroid-disease screenings, educational information/seminars, and thyroid physician referrals.

Publications

American Thyroid Association
www.thyroid.org

A professional organization of physicians and scientists dedicated to scientific research on the thyroid. The association refers the public to member physicians in their geographic area on request. Publishes a quarterly newsletter and patient-education brochures.

National Graves' Disease Foundation
www.ngdf.org

Provides medical information, referral, and resource information to patients; aids in the development of support groups; provides professional education through lectures and forums; and sponsors, develops, participates in, and supports research on Graves' disease. Publishes a quarterly newsletter and patient-education brochures.

Thyroid Foundation of America, Inc.
www.tsh.org

Provides public-education programs, patient information, and support. Refers patients to qualified endocrinologists. Publishes a quarterly newsletter and information brochures.

The Thyroid Society for Education and Research
www.the-thyroid-society.org

Pursues the prevention, treatment, and cure of thyroid disease and fosters patient, physician, and community education. Publishes a quarterly newsletter and patient-education brochures.

Researching test results
going online for test guidelines

Lab tests become a key part of your treatment when you have a thyroid condition. That's because your thyroid-hormone levels need to be checked periodically to make sure you are getting the correct amounts. It's natural to be confused and scared when told the results of your tests. One way to overcome your fears is to learn about the nature of thyroid tests. The Internet can offer some excellent instructions on the fine art of understanding thyroid tests.

Try Lab Tests Online (**www.labtestsonline.org**). Here you can find a reasoned discussion of what labs set out to measure, how they do it, and what the results mean. You will want to read up on the significance of reference ranges before you try to make sense of any lab results you may have. Reference ranges are like pulse rates—they vary and are tough to pin down. All kinds of factors can play into what constitutes a "normal" range, including the age and sex of the patient. Labs attempt to establish a range of normal levels from lots of samples—your results will show the normal range the lab expects. But "normal" is a bit of a sliding scale. Different labs may have different ranges, and according to Lab Tests Online, very few lab tests have published and nationally agreed-upon reference ranges across the board (see pages 204–205).

Two other excellent resources for understanding thyroid tests come from the government publication Medline's medical encyclopedia and the nonprofit site EndocrineWeb. At Medline, **http://medlineplus.org,** enter the test name in the search box (typing something as simple as "T4 test" will do it) and read the article. For EndocrineWeb's page, go straight to **www.endocrineweb.com/tests.html**.

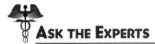

My doctor said my TSH was at the low end of normal, and that I was fine. But I don't feel fine. I still have many symptoms of hypothyroidism. Am I okay?

An astute physician will check out T_3 and T_4 levels if the TSH is low normal and your symptoms are still bothering you. It could be that you have **subclinical hypothyroidism**—a condition where the thyroid function is on the low edge of normal. If the patient has some hypothyroid symptoms or high cholesterol, then the new wisdom is to treat subclinical hypothyroidism with thyroid-hormone supplements. To get the best medical care, a physician needs to factor in clinical examination and an assessment of your symptoms. That said, if your TSH and other thyroid hormone levels are all normal, then your doctor should rule out thyroid disease and look for other possible causes of your symptoms.

News flash

It may be helpful to know that as of January 2003, the American Association of Clinical Endocrinologists has announced new guidelines for the TSH test. Previously, normal for TSH was between 0.5 and 5.0 micro units per milliliter of blood. The new guidelines are 0.3 and 3.0.

Researching doctors
go online to find the right medical help

The Internet is also very useful in helping you locate doctors in your area who are thyroid specialists. This is especially crucial if you want a second opinion about your thyroid condition or if you are moving to a new town and want to find a thyroid specialist before you arrive.

There are several general doctor sites that are helpful. You can go to the American Medical Association Web page, **www.ama-assn.org**. Click on their Doctor Finder tab and you can find thyroid specialists in your state and region. You can also try the Doctor Directory online. Go to **www.doctordirectory.com,** and you will see listings of doctors by specialty as well as region. Another approach is to go to the dedicated thyroid Web sites and use their doctor services. Try these sites:

> **www.thyroid.org/resources/patients/specialists.php3**
>
> **www.aace.com/memsearch.php**
> (under Specialty, select Thyroid Dysfunction)
>
> **www.endocrineweb.com/docsearch/**

Doctors and Internet-Savvy Patients

Some doctors get alarmed when patients come in with reams of print-outs from the Internet. While it's true that some sites cannot be trusted, a number of medical Web sites have a formal panel of medical advisers—just like the physicians' favorite reading material, *The New England Journal of Medicine*. Your goal is to enter into a dialogue with your doctor about your health. Use the information you get off the Internet as a springboard for discussion.

Researching Alternative Therapies

The Internet is also an excellent resource when you would like to find out about alternative therapies. For more on complementary therapies, see pages 97–108. For a good use of your time, try a pinpointed search. Go to **www.ask.com** and type in "thyroid" and the name of the therapy you are interested in. You will be taken to related Web pages. Another approach is to check out some tried-and-true alternative sites. Here are a few:.

Dr. Andrew Weil is an AMA-trained doctor who has been one of the leading forces behind the holistic-medicine movement. His site, **www.drweil.com,** covers all sorts of disorders and offers advice on various types of alternative treatments. When you type in your particular disorder, you may find that the good doctor has some alternative-therapy advice that can help.

Another useful site is Healthplus. This site is composed of a consortium of alternative therapies. Visit it to learn about any of the various therapies available, be it yoga or light therapy. It also has a tab for finding practitioners. Go to **www.healthplusweb.com.**

Another site, HealthWorld Online at **www.healthy.net,** has a referral service that will point you to doctors who practice "integrative medicine," which means they combine traditional AMA medicine with alternative treatments.

Keeping useful records
Create your own research portfolio

It's easy to get lost when you first go online to learn about your new condition. There are all sorts of sites out there. One way to make sense of it all is to keep notes on where you travel on the Internet highway. In fact, you can use your computer to chart your journey. Here's how:

Bookmark important pages. Great, you have just hit the mother lode of information—a page with tons of handy links and lots of good solid information. Instead of stopping to write down the name of the site, save time and bookmark it! Every Web browser has the ability to let you save the names of favorite Web pages. All you have to do is be on the Web page you want to note, go up to the toolbar, and click on the correct tab that will tell your computer to make a snapshot of the site. In Internet Explorer, click on Favorites; in America Online, click on Favorite Places; and in Netscape, click on Bookmarks. To access that favorite Web page, all you need to do is look through your list of favorite sites or bookmarks and click on it.

Print out important information. When you find a page with a lot of relevant information on it, print it out and file it in your health journal (see page 14). Just get a three-hole punch so you can put your printouts tidily away into your binder. As the number of printouts grows, you can categorize them by topic: medicine, specialists, alternative therapies, and so on. This will make it easier to find the information.

Save time and paper

You don't have to print a whole Web page. Highlight just the bit that interests you, click on File, then Print, and in the Print box, click Selection. Then click on the OK button or "Apply" and you'll have a nice short printout.

—

Evaluating Web Sites

Not all the information on the Web is accurate. Before you start thickening up your health journal, make sure the Web pages you want to copy are providing solid information. The sites you find may contain outdated facts, misinformation, poor research, urban legends, propaganda, and outright lies. How can you tell what's good and what is not? Use this checklist.

1. Check the date. In a book or newspaper, you can always see the publication date—so you know whether the information is current. On the Web, not every page carries the publication date. The better medical sites do. If you don't see a date, don't trust any figures the page calls "current."

2. Check out the source. Most articles online have bylines stating the writer's name. If you have not heard of the writer or you don't know his or her reputation, feed the name into a search engine (see page 85) and see who else carries the byline. A good medical paper always backs up its statements with sources and bibliographies. Check any article for sources and links to other sites.

3. Check out the publisher. Look at the Web address of any article you are evaluating. Is it a name you recognize—a well-known clinic or foundation or government site? If not, look around for a link labeled "About this site" or something like that, and see who is behind it all.

4. Don't be put off by advertising. Advertising is a fact of life on the Web. One exception: If a site seems to be selling something in its articles, move on. You cannot trust advertorials on television, so don't trust your health to them online.

Online support
check out online chat rooms

Having a chronic health condition is stressful, to say the least. This is especially true with thyroid disorders, whose symptoms can really wreak havoc on your life. For some, the weight gain is very difficult to manage, while for others, the fatigue and anxiety are the hardest to deal with. For still others the process of finding the right treatment is the most taxing. It can take months, sometimes years, to settle on the right dosage of medication. For all these reasons, finding support from like-minded souls who know your pain and suffering firsthand can be comforting. Again, the Internet can help.

There are a few sites that offer **chat rooms** (online forums where messages can be typed in and responded to in real time). Another option is message boards. Here you can post a message or a question to the board and ask for feedback. Check back a few days later and you will no doubt find several helpful answers.

There are rules set forth by most virtual communities. Some ask that you stick to the medical aspects of your condition only, while others invite you to talk about anything. Use your judgment and see what you find.

Online thyroid chat rooms and message boards can be found at **www.thyroid-info.com.**

A friend in need, a friend indeed

When I was first diagnosed with Graves' disease and complete-ly falling apart, I spent a lot of late nights online, looking for information on treatments, research . . . anything. And instead, I made a friend online who also has Graves'.

At first we chatted a lot about our illness in general in a public chat area. As we got to know each other better, we began exchanging private e-mails on a pretty regular basis. It is so helpful to know that I can e-mail her whenever I run into a health crisis. Sure, my friends and family are supportive, but there is something really special about sharing your ups and downs with someone who is right there in the trenches with you. Moreover, she has helped with advice on little practical everyday things, like resting in the evenings and learning to say no and mean it when I'm asked to volunteer in the kids' school. She has also encouraged me to be more assertive with my doctor.

She lives in California, and I'm not sure we will ever meet in person. For now, I'm grateful for her kindness, caring, and wisdom. I'm so glad she and I had the chance to connect.

—Cindy C., Miami, FL

Helpful resources

After Any Diagnosis
by Carol Svec

Thyroid Manager
http://www.thyroidmanager.org/
thyroidbook.htm
A book written by two dozen M.D.'s
from across the world. It's thorough,
heavy going at times but truly indis-
pensable stuff when you are ready to
really dig in. The authors and editors continuously review thyroid literature and select new material to
update the site.

**The Merck Manual of Diagnosis
and Therapy**
http://www.merck.com/pubs/
mmanual/section2/sec2.htm
Click on Chapter 8 to read the thyroid section of this vast pharmaceutical company's manual—but only if
you are ready for a lot of biochemistry. This publication is by and
large for pharmaceutical experts,
and although it's written clearly, it
does not shy away from polysylla-
bles—there are a lot of chemical
names floating around here!

eMedicine's Endocrinology
http://www.emedicine.com/med/
endocrinology.htm
eMedicine is a textbook example of
a trustworthy resource. Each article
is dated, so you know how recent
the information is, you get to read
the name and credentials of the
writer and board of editors that

reviewed the article, and every article has an extensive bibliography.
The articles themselves read like
encyclopedia entries, with sections
covering the background, clinical
symptoms, treatments, labs, procedures, medication, and follow-up for
each condition. To get access to a lot
of the good stuff, you need to regis-
ter at the site. You don't need to pay
or give much information to regis-
ter—just your e-mail address and
details of your level of education.

The Health Resource
www.theheathresource.com
Tel: 800 949-0090
You don't have to search the
Internet yourself. There are a number of companies that offer this
service for a fee. One such company,
called The Health Resource, will do
extensive Internet research com-
plilation that is customized to your
diagnosis. The company's Internet
specialists will then comb through
the Internet and other sources and
locate medical articles geared
toward your specific situation,
including mainstream, experimental, and alternative treatments along
with top specialists. In a week to 10
days, you will receive a hard copy of
their findings in a bound booklet,
complete with glossary. Prices range
from $150 to $400.

CHAPTER 6

Complementary Therapies

Weighing your alternatives
identifying your needs

For some, living with a chronic illness is the first time they have ever taken their health seriously enough to reflect on their lifestyle and make healthy changes. That's good. As the saying goes: to live a long life, get a good disease. But for others, having a chronic illness, even one as nominal as a minor thyroid disorder, is just one more stressor that they have to deal with. Somewhere in all this lies a happy medium—a place for stress relief and a restored sense of well-being. Enter the world of complementary medicine.

What will help you depends on what troubles you the most about your illness. If you are frightened or angry or depressed, you may benefit from techniques that emphasize the mind-body connection, such as meditation, biofeedback, or exercise that requires mental focus, such as yoga or tai chi. Complementary therapies are often called "alternative medicine." But to call something an "alternative" suggests that you do either one or the other. It's more useful and more accurate to think of these treatments as supplemental or complementary to your standard treatment. Just be aware that most complementary therapies have yet to be validated by scientific studies.

If you decide to explore complementary therapies, be certain to discuss your plans and discoveries with your doctor. It's essential that your doctor knows what you are doing in order to be able to judge how it might interact with your standard treatment.

Use your common sense

◆ **Research what's available.** Support groups can be helpful sources of information on symptom relief. Ask the research librarian at your library to help you find one in your town. Or do an Internet search using the name of your illness plus the name of the therapy you want to explore.

◆ **Avoid thinking that because something is "natural" it is benign.** Many of the so-called natural substances touted by alternative healers have not been tested, let alone approved, by the F.D.A. Personal experiences and anecdotal evidence do not make them "safe." Be especially wary of taking any products that are sold directly by a healer. Talk with your doctor first before you try anything.

◆ **Stay alert to how you are feeling.** It's tempting to think that you "feel lousy all the time." In truth, you probably have good days and bad days. The more you know about what makes you feel better or worse, the more you can use that knowledge to improve your well-being. Review your health journal (see page 14).

◆ **Bear the expense in mind.** Complementary treatments can cost as much as standard methods—or more, given that many are not covered by insurance plans. Be as frank about your finances as you are about your physical condition. Some practitioners may be willing to negotiate their fees.

◆ **Above all, do not fall for the notion that if the therapy fails, you have failed.** Nothing, not even antibiotics, works equally well for everyone. Give the new therapy a fair trial—some can take a while to show a benefit—but if you are not being helped, give it up and try something else. Or try another person who practices the same therapy; that person may have an insight that makes all the difference.

Massage and bodywork
the lowdown on getting a rubdown

The stress response causes our muscles to tighten. Not surprisingly, chronic stress can lead to chronic muscle fatigue and pain. One way to mitigate the stress in your life is through bodywork. *Bodywork* is the catchall term for a range of physical therapies that involve manipulation of the body. As with other complementary therapies, bodywork is very helpful at relieving stress-related symptoms.

People who practice therapeutic massage generally avoid the words *masseuse* and *masseur* and instead call themselves "massage therapists." Their ads will state that they practice therapeutic, medical, or sports massage; in states where the practice is regulated by the government, the abbreviation LMT (licensed massage therapist) may follow the person's name. Another string of letters to look for is NCTMB. This means that the therapist has received at least 500 hours of training and has passed a qualifying exam administered by the National Certification Board for Therapeutic Massage and Bodywork. In states where massage is a licensed health practice, your insurance company may reimburse some of the costs.

In general, "massage" means Swedish massage or Shiatsu (see page 101), and "bodywork" encompasses a wide range of other physically based therapies. Another distinction, albeit a fine one, is that massage is often limited to physical manipulation, while bodywork encompasses the idea that the body is also composed of energy fields and channels and that blocked energy causes or exacerbates disease.

The different practices vary in intensity and therapeutic benefits; almost all of them can be successfully administered while you are clothed. Also, different therapists have different "touches"—some work gently, others work vigorously. Ask the therapist how much discomfort you may experience as an inherent part of the treatment; if the therapist is working too deeply, speak up.

Here's a look at some popular bodywork therapies. To get more information, or for help in locating a practitioner, see Helpful resources, page 108.

Swedish massage Originally intended to help improve blood circulation and encourage drainage of the lymph system, this technique uses gliding, kneading, tapping, and vibrating strokes for gentle or penetrating muscle massage. It is especially helpful for tension relief and relaxation.

Myofascial therapy This is a general term for a number of techniques that manipulate soft tissue—muscle fibers (myo-) and the connective tissue that holds muscle fibers in place (fascia)—to relieve "trigger points," localized areas that are either painful themselves or provoke pain in other areas.

Rolfing Developed by Ida P. Rolf, a biochemist, who called the process "Structural Integration." It is a form of deep manipulation of the body's soft tissues. Practitioners are trained and certified by the Rolf Institute in Colorado.

Shiatsu (acupressure) A component of traditional Chinese medicine. Practitioners use fingertip pressure on specific points along the body's energy channels to release blocked energy.

Cranio-Sacral Therapy (CST) Practitioners gently manipulate the skull, the sacrum, and the nerve endings in the scalp. It can be helpful for back and neck pain and headache. Practitioners are trained and certified by the Upledger Institute in Florida.

The Trager Approach Nonintrusive massage and movement reeducation that focuses on integrating the mind and body to relieve anxiety. Practitioners are trained and certified by the Trager Institute in Ohio.

Stress management
teaching your mind to soothe your body

After a few months of taking Synthroid, your hormone levels are normal but you are still feeling anxious and stressed out. Not only do you feel bad, you feel bad about feeling bad. What can you do? Once you have ruled out depression and anxiety disorders as well as an incorrrect dosage of Synthroid, you will probably have to learn to incorporate some stress-management techniques into your life.

Learning to relax sounds counterintuitive, even insultingly simplistic. Relaxing should be instinctive, and under the best of circumstances it is. But being diagnosed with a chronic illness is a life-changing, anxiety-provoking experience, and it's easy to get so bound up with stress that you don't realize how stressed you are. Practitioners of the so-called mind-body modalities teach you to be more conscious of stress and give you practical things to do about it. Again, it may seem counterintuitive to focus on stress—after all, we are hardwired to recoil from pain and culturally pro-grammed to pull up our socks and get on with things. But with proper guidance, stress management can yield enormous benefits, not just physi-cally but also mentally, emotionally, and spiritually. When you feel better, you are better.

Biofeedback was one of the earliest stress-management techniques to gain credence with medical doctors, perhaps because it uses computers to audit measurable physiological functions. In a typical session you may have a few small sensors attached to your head or heart. The sensors measure your brain waves, skin temperature, heart rate, level of muscle tension, and blood pressure. These sensors are connected to a computer that displays this information in graph form on a computer screen. As you watch the screen, you can see your heart rate slowing and your muscles relaxing. This improves blood flow, which raises the temperature of your hands. (People who suffer from "cold body syndrome" feel that this alone is worth the price of admission.) The computer screen gives you ongoing feedback about your physical condition. You can actually see how changing your mind changes your body. People usually need about 12 sessions to master the technique. Imagine learning how to feel warm again or stress-free simply by using your mind. The National Institutes of Health has issued a statement saying that biofeedback is an underutilized therapy, considering how effective it is clinically.

Relaxation therapy encompasses a wide range of techniques designed to reduce stress and tension. Some of the more popular ones are:

◆ **Progressive muscle relaxation** You do this by systematically tensing and relaxing the muscles in each part of your body. While sitting comfortably or lying down, inhale and clench your facial muscles, hold the tension for a moment, then exhale and relax those muscles. Do the same thing with your shoulders, one arm, then the other—and so on through your body until you get to your toes. When you're done, stay quietly where you are and breathe normally for a few minutes.

◆ **Guided imagery** The idea here is to imagine a peaceful place and put yourself in the scene. This is usually done with a partner who provides the "guidance" by describing the scene, but you can do all the imagining yourself or listen to a narrated audiotape or to soothing music or environmental sounds, such as birdsong or ocean waves.

◆ **Deep breathing** Taking a few minutes each day to practice slow, deep breathing can relieve muscle pain and light-headedness, plus improve mental acuity. All you need to do is stand, sit, or lie still; slowly inhale for five seconds, then exhale slowly and completely for another five seconds. Repeat this for 10 breaths and it should help trigger the relaxation response.

Meditation
using the metaphysical to help the physical

Studies show that regular meditation can lower blood pressure, relieve chronic pain, and reduce cortisol levels, a measure of the body's stress. It may also help if you suffer from frequent, severe headaches. It can also help teach your body how to relax. Dr. Herbert Benson, a cardiologist, did a great deal of research on meditation and found that it can actually lower autonomic nervous system activity, which means that meditation allows your body to truly relax. Dr. Benson dubbed this phenomenon "the relaxation response."

How can something so simple as meditation do such wonders? There is no hard answer. Most practitioners say it works because it transports both the body and the mind into a uniquely unified state. As Dr. Lawrence Edwards, a meditation teacher in Bedford Hills, New York, explains, "Meditation is a transformation process. Over time, meditation profoundly changes the mind and body, allowing you to more quickly access a sense of peace and inner freedom. Every time you meditate, you are increasing the reservoir of meditative power that you can tap into during stressful or challenging moments."

There are a number of different meditation techniques to consider. Some focus on the breath, while others use a mantra (a sacred word or phrase that you repeat over and over again). The goal is the same: to focus your attention away from the thoughts whirling around inside your head. The repetition of breath or mantra helps calm the mind down so it can enter into a meditative state. Unlike guided imagery (see page 103), classic meditation does not involve talking or music, but it may be helpful to light a scented candle or burn incense. That's because your mind will associate the fragrance with "it's time to settle down," which can help ease your transition into the practice. It's also helpful to meditate at the same time every day and for the same amount of time, even if it's only a few minutes.

How to Meditate

Find a place you can sit quietly without interruptions for 20 minutes.

Sit comfortably, but keep your back erect—this will help support alertness and open breathing. (You can meditate lying down if you are not able to sit up.)

Set a timer for 15 to 20 minutes.

Close your eyes and bring your attention to your breathing. Focus on the movement of your diaphragm as you inhale and exhale.

As you settle into this quiet breathing, you can repeat your mantra or any word you wish silently to yourself. You can use the traditional Sanskrit words *Om Namah Shivaya,* or say a phrase of your own choosing, or simply the words "one, two, three, four."

When your mind begins to wander, as it inevitably will, just gently return your focus to your breath or mantra. This pattern of wandering and returning is the beginning of teaching your mind to let go of its worries.

When the timer buzzes, notice how at peace you feel. Open your eyes and stretch.

Choose a regular time and place to meditate. Start by meditating for 20 minutes three times a week. Stay with it.

Yoga, the "mindful" exercise
using yoga to help your thyroid problem

The goals of yogic exercise are to teach you to pay attention to your body as you breathe and exercise. You want to coordinate your breath with your movements. For this reason, some people consider yoga a "mindful" exercise, a form of meditation in motion. But how does that help your health? Studies have shown that yoga promotes mental and emotional clarity; improves balance, flexibility, strength, and stamina; relieves chronic muscle aches; eliminates stress; and helps to regulate your metabolism.

There are variations in the way yoga is taught. Some classes are slow paced, others are as lively as a step-aerobics class. Typically, yoga classes can be paid for one at a time, or in sets of 5 or 10 with a discounted price. If you are curious but skeptical, ask to observe a class; you should be able to do this for free. Class lengths vary; a midday class may be 30 or 45 minutes, but an evening class may be 60 or 90 minutes long—and priced accordingly. Shop around until you find something that suits you. A number of books, videotapes, and DVDs are available that feature beginning exercises that you can do at home.

Qigong and Tai Chi

According to the National Qigong Association, qigong is "an ancient Chinese health-care system that integrates physical postures, breathing techniques, and focused intention." Pronounced CHEE gung—and sometimes spelled "Chi Kung"— the word means "cultivating energy." Tai chi is a form of qigong; both are gentle exercise routines that promote vitality. Tai chi is also a martial art, and the sequence of gestures used in it helps to prepare the person, mentally and physically, for fighting. Both qigong and tai chi consist of a specific series of dancelike gestures that are performed in a specific sequence. The sequence of gestures is called a form, and there are long and short forms of the exercises. In tai chi, the short form takes about 10 minutes to complete; it's a bit longer for qiqong. Practitioners of the form say that the sense of vitality you feel afterward will last throughout the day.

FIRST PERSON INSIGHTS

Finally, help for my aching back

A friend recommended that I see a massage therapist in town, to alleviate some lower-back pain that started after I was gardening. I met the practitioner in her office and we talked a bit about my back pain and the kind of work I do throughout the day. She showed me two stretches that would help allieviate some tension. She told me she would leave the room for a few minutes so I could undress down to my underwear and get on the table, facedown, and pull the sheet over me. After a few minutes, she knocked on the door and asked if I was ready. I said yes and she came in and lowered the lights, turned on some soothing music, and poured a bit of body oil in her hands. For the next hour, she worked on my back. Once I got over being nervous, I found myself relaxing. When she hit a troublesome spot, she asked me to breathe along with her while she worked on it. It was really amazing, but by the end of the session, my back felt great.

—Eric L., Austin, TX

Helpful resources

**National Center for
Complementary and Alternative
Medicine (NCCAM)
National Institutes of Health**
Bethesda, MD 20892
**Tel: 888 644-6226
http://nccam.nih.gov**
This government agency provides
information about and sponsors
research in complementary
therapies.

**American Council on Science
and Health**
1995 Broadway, 2nd floor
New York, NY 10023-5860
**Tel: 212 362-7044
fax: 212 362-4919
www.acsh.org**

www.alternativehealing.org
This site is full of advice and expla-
nations about every kind of alternative treatment under the sun.

www.quackwatch.com
The organization Quack Watch
keeps tabs on fringe alternative
therapies.

CHAPTER 7

Putting *Your* Team *Together*

Your primary-care doctor
know what to expect from your GP

If you are like most people with a thyroid condition, it was probably your primary-care doctor or internist who raised the red flag and ordered tests that confirmed your illness. This, however, is the best-case scenario; the worst case is one in which your primary doctor misdiagnosed your thyroid condition and it took another doctor or perhaps a specialist to get you back on track.

Does this mean your primary-care doctor is unqualified? Not necessarily. Most primary-care doctors are generalists, so they usually take a "symptom by symptom" approach to treating complaints. Moreover, they can only rely on the information they get from their patients. Alas, most patients don't know how to articulate their symptoms, so the doctor often gets incomplete or misleading information. This is especially true of thyroid symptoms, which so often mimic classic stress overload or depression (see page 12).

If you have been diagnosed and are happy with your current primary-care doctor, then by all means stick with this doctor. Even after you have been referred to a specialist, you will still need to have a regular doctor on hand. Just because you have a thyroid disorder does not mean you will be spared an occasional bout with the flu or a sinus infection—you'll need the help of your primary-care doctor, not to mention that yearly physical check-up. A good primary-care physician should act as the "gatekeeper" who manages your general health care and knows when to send you on to a more specialized doctor.

Working with your doctor is a two-way street

Developing a good relationship with your primary-care doctor requires effort on both sides. Just as you have rights and responsibilities as a patient, your doctor has certain rights and responsibilities. And as with any relationship, the doctor-patient one rests on respect and trust. These are some of your rights in the doctor-patient relationship:

- To be fully informed about your diagnosis, prognosis, and treatment
- To have a say in decisions affecting your health
- To have all your questions and concerns dealt with
- To have your medical records released only with your consent
- To have reasonable access to your doctor
- To be told about the costs and risks of treatment
- To change doctors, request a referral, or get a second opinion
- To be seen within a reasonable amount of time
- To be told about how a test or procedure works, how much it costs, and what the alternatives and risks are before consenting to treatment

In return, doctors have a right to be treated with common courtesy, to be allowed enough time to make a diagnosis, to have their advice followed carefully, and to be notified in a timely manner if you must cancel or change an appointment.

When should you get a second opinion?

There are several instances in which you are justified in seeking a second opinion: if the diagnosis is uncertain or life-threatening; if the tests or treatment are controversial, experimental, or risky; if you do not like the doctor's approach; if you have questions about the doctor's competency. Do not be afraid that by asking for a second opinion you are offending your doctor. Most doctors want their patients to be proactive about their care and are more than happy to recommend other specialists for them to see.

Your endocrinologist
front-line specialists in thyroid disorders

Although most internists are more than capable of treating everyday thyroid disorders, difficult cases usually require a thyroid specialist. In those instances, you will be referred to an **endocrinologist,** a doctor who specializes in diseases of the glands or endocrine system. This means that in addition to medical school, the doctor has spent several years studying endocrinology and has passed the state medical tests in that specialty and been admitted to the medical board as a specialist.

How does this translate into treatment? Most likely, a specialist will be even busier than a regular doctor, will be harder to make appointments with, and will charge more for your appointment. She may also use more medical jargon and treat you more like a "case" than a person. But there are certainly exceptions to this, and there are many warm and caring specialists out there.

Just in case, though, when you visit a thyroid specialist you need to be ready to present your "case" as quickly, accurately, and thoroughly as possible. As with a visit to your GP, make the most of this visit by preparing questions beforehand, taking notes during your visit, and requesting any relevant literature from the specialist. All of this will go a long way toward making any unfamiliar concepts easier to grasp.

Finding a Thyroid Specialist

Mary Shomon's highly informative Web site on thyroid disorders has a database that allows you to search for thyroid specialists by state or preferred treatment. Check out this link:
www.thyroid-info.com/topdrs/index.htm

Finding the right endocrinologist

Just because you have been referred to an endocrinologist does not mean that this doctor is a specialist in thyroid conditions. Sometimes an endocrinologist will be a specialist in diabetes or fertility medicine. However, this does not mean she cannot treat run-of-the-mill thyroid problems.

To find out if an endocrinologist is right for you, you should get answers to the following questions:

1. How many people with thyroid problems does the doctor treat every day? If the number is under 3, this doctor is probably not focusing on thyroid disorders. Most endocrinologists see 10 thyroid patients a day. You should be working with one who treats that many.

2. What kinds of diagnostic tests does the doctor use? Most endocrinologists rely on the "thyroid panel" (TSH, total T_4 and T_3). Other tests they may use are the radioactive iodine uptake test (RAI) and the thyroperoxidase antibody test (anti-TPO).

3. What kinds of medication does the doctor usually prescribe? If the doctor is a big believer in a synthetic hormone medicine such as Synthroid and you are interested in trying natural thyroid medication, this may not be the doctor for you.

Putting your team together
who you will need, and why

Because the thyroid gland controls so many bodily functions, from circulation to digestion, thyroid disorders can impact your health in a number of different ways. Thyroid disorders can affect your heart, your eyes, your digestion—not to mention your mental health. This is why the list of doctors you might need includes more than just your primary-care physician and an endocrinologist. Ideally, your primary-care doctor will refer you to any specialists you will need. It's very important that all of your doctors communicate to each other about your care. Your primary-care physician or endocrinologist should be able to coordinate that communication.

Questions to Ask Specialists

Bear in mind, it's rare that you will speak to the doctor before your first appointment. However, his or her staff should be able to answer these simple questions:

How long has the doctor been specializing in thyroid-related disorders? Some endrocrinologists specialize in diabetes and do very little work with thyroid patients.

How much does the doctor charge for a consultation? Does his or her office accept your insurance? This is another important question, especially since a number of health insurers don't pay for a second opinion. Know up front what the cost is before you walk in the door.

What type of information does the doctor need to see on that first consultation? Having the right information on hand can make or break a visit with a specialist. Be sure you have exactly what the doctor will need to best evaluate your case (see pages 118–119).

Medical specialists you may need

Ophthalmologist People with Graves' disease often develop thyroid eye disease (TED). If you develop problems with your eye muscles that require surgery, the ophthalmologist may send you to a strabismologist, an eye muscle specialist.

Radiation oncologist If you need to undergo radiation or chemotherapy for thyroid cancer, this doctor will be in charge of treatment.

Nuclear-medicine specialist This is the doctor who administers the radioactive iodine test or administers radioactive iodine as treatment.

Cardiologist Both hyperthyroidism and hypothyroidism can cause or exacerbate heart problems.

Gynecologist or andrologist Women whose thyroid condition is affecting their fertility or libido are referred to a gynecologist, men to an andrologist.

Internist This is the umbrella term for doctors who handle disorders of the internal organs. Kidney and liver problems can be related to thyroid illness. Most primary-care doctors are internists.

Dietitian Weight gain is a common problem for hypothyroid people, and a dietitian or nutritionist can develop a "thyroid healthy" diet to help.

Gerontologist Since thyroid problems in the elderly (especially women) can manifest themselves very differently than in younger people, you may be referred to this doctor if you are over 50.

Pediatrician A doctor who specializes in the medical care of children.

Creating a health portfolio
organizing your medical records

There is a lot of paperwork involved when you have a chronic illness. There are medical forms, test results, treatment plans, prescription plans, and myriad insurance forms. Because you will probably end up working with different doctors, you need to find a way to organize your records so each doctor has easy access to information about your health. You can do this by keeping records of your tests and treatments in a "health portfolio."

Your health portfolio should contain the "public" information about your disorder, separate from your health journal (see pages 14–15) which, depending on its contents, you may or may not want to share with your doctor. Separate each topic into its own section, for example:

◆ Thyroid test results: TSH blood tests, FNA test, RAI tests, and so on.
◆ Treatments: notes on thyroid treatments. Include dates of doctor's visits and what happened during the visit treatment-wise.
◆ Results of other non–thyroid-related tests: blood pressure, angiograms, CT scans, MRI reports.
◆ Other illnesses you may have and the treatment.
◆ Medication: Include start/stop dates, dosage levels, effects, plus any information on allergies you may have.
◆ Your family health history.
◆ Contact information: List name, hours, phone numbers, receptionists' names for your doctor, pharmacist, and lab/treatment facility.

Preparing for an appointment

With your health portfolio in hand, it's a lot easier to turn your doctor's appointments into effective meetings. In fact, some people with chronic illnesses advise preparing for a doctor's appointment as you would for a business meeting. That means thinking about issues you want to discuss. Jot them down so you will not forget. Your goal is to take an active role in your appointment. Here are some guidelines:

1. Educate yourself about the latest research, diagnoses, theories, and treatments, and be ready to discuss them with your doctor.

2. If you come across any unfamiliar terminology, look it up or make a list to ask your doctor.

3. Prepare a list of questions ahead of time.

4. Keep your health journal (see page 14) up-to-date and review it before the visit to remind yourself of any development you want to discuss.

5. Be on time. If you are early, review your notes.

6. If you are anxious, bring a friend or family member for support (see page 124). Make sure this support person knows your concerns ahead of time. If you are worried that you will forget what the doctor is telling you, ask your support person to take notes for you.

7. During the visit, be as professional as possible. Keep in mind that you have the right to question the doctor's recommendations, diagnoses, and prescriptions.

8. Always ask questions if you don't understand what your doctor is telling you. It is quite all right to ask your doctor to explain your lab-test results.

9. At the end of the visit, summarize any new treatments or prescriptions. Put any new test results in your health portfolio.

10. Ask for copies of the results of any medical tests.

Using your health journal
looking for clues in your health journal

While it's true that living with a chronic disease means you will need to make some changes, it does not mean your quality of life must change for the worse. In fact, with some smart planning and a little bit of knowledge, you can learn to manage your thyroid disease like a pro. Some even say that learning how to manage their illness taught them invaluable life lessons. So how do you manage a chronic illness? Take a tip from the CEOs of the business world—all you really need is good information and a good team.

Your good information is right at your fingertips. Literally. All you need to do is pay attention to your body and track your symptoms in your health journal (see page 14). Before a doctor's visit, read through the last three months and see if there are any new patterns developing.

Your next step is to create a good support team that can effectively use the "inside" information you have been carefully noting. This means looking for people who are in tune with you and make you feel comfortable. Consider them members of your own personal board of directors, who can help you manage your illness like a pro. With the right information and the right team, you are ready for anything.

Looking for patterns

From time to time, it's a good idea to review your health journal. You are looking for any unusual occurrence, as well as any patterns. Again, it's important to bear in mind that learning to listen to and observe your body is hard. It takes time to learn to pay attention to it. Reviewing your journal will keep you in the habit of thinking about your health. Things to look for:

- Sleep patterns. Are you sleeping more or less? Is your sleep restful or fitful?
- Diet and digestion patterns. Are you craving any foods? Having difficulty digesting certain foods? Eating more or less? At different times of the day?
- Accounts of any life events that seem to be affecting your health, plus a record of your daily stress level.
- Emotional mood patterns. This one is hard. You are looking for patterns of feelings; for example, feelings of sadness striking every afternoon—may reveal a blood-sugar problem.
- Record of symptoms, including date, time, type, duration, and intensity. Also note any precipitating factors and what seems to make symptoms worsen or go away.

Thyroid surgeons
when you need thyroid surgery

If your GP or endocrinologist has prescribed surgery to remove your thyroid gland or thyroid nodules, you will be referred to an endocrine surgeon, a head and neck surgeon, or an otolaryngologist (also known as an ENT or an ear, nose, and throat doctor). You might also be referred to a plastic surgeon.

As with other doctors, you will need to ask some important questions before you go through surgery. When you meet with the surgeon, ask questions about her educational background and experience. You will want to know how often the surgeon does this type of operation, if any of the doctor's patients have had any serious complications, and if any have died during the procedure (very uncommon).

If you would like a second opinion after meeting with the surgeon referred by your doctor, where do you look? One place to start is **www.endocrinesurgeons.org,** where you can search for surgeons by state. Look for a surgeon who is a true thyroid specialist and has done thyroid operations before, because some endocrine surgeons focus only on the pancreas or other glands, while some head and neck surgeons may work only on cranial disorders. An ENT may be a specialist in only vocal-cord surgery, for example, and not thyroid surgery.

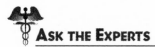

Ask the Experts

I'm having a thyroidectomy. How pronounced will the scar be?

In terms of your appearance, your thyroid surgery is likely to leave a very small, almost invisible scar, which will be well hidden by the natural fold of skin on your neck. In some cases, the wound may become infected postsurgery, which can cause some scarring, but this is very rare.

My surgeon has told me that removing my thyroid nodules will be as simple as taking out my tonsils, but I'm not convinced.

Your doctor may be exaggerating a little, but in truth the risks of complications from thyroid surgery are pretty slim. About 1 percent of people will have some damage to the nerves of the voice box or slight damage to the parathyroid glands (the glands that sit atop the thyroid gland), which might lead to tingling or numbness of the mouth, hands, and feet.

I've been told about this new type of endoscopic surgery to remove nodules. How safe is it?

Recently, doctors have been experimenting with a new surgical procedure, called **endoscopic thyroid surgery,** to remove nodules. This procedure is much less invasive than traditional thyroid surgery. It involves inserting a very small tube in the neck and using carbon monoxide gas to slightly inflate the area. Then the doctor inserts another tube with a scalpel edge to remove the nodule. Although this type of surgery takes a little longer, the scar is even less noticeable and patients can usually return to their normal schedule more quickly.

Your pharmacist
the "safety net" in managing your illness

Because you will probably be taking thyroid medication for life, developing a relationship with your pharmacist is a good idea. This way, your pharmacist can act as a "safety net" in managing your prescriptions, not only for your thyroid medicine but for any adverse drug interactions with other medications you may take as well.

That's why the best strategy is to work with one pharmacist—someone whose experience and background you trust and who takes the time to answer your questions. Also, using one pharmacist will make it easier to keep your medication records up-to-date. If you use the more impersonal drug chains for your pharmaceutical needs, then make sure to do a drug check with your doctor at least once a year.

When you pick up your prescription, ask about the expiration dates of your medicine. This is extremely important to know, because many thyroid-medication manufacturers do not list the expiration date on the label. It's also important because your pharmacist may have had the medication on the shelf for quite a while before dispensing it to you.

Finally, double-check with your pharmacist about when and how to take your medications, and make sure these instructions match what is printed on the bottle.

Keep it handy

Always keep a list in your wallet or purse of the medicines you are taking and the dosages. In case of an emergency, this list will prove invaluable.

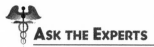

ASK THE EXPERTS

I have a prescription for three months of Synthroid with four repeats, and my pharmacist offered to fill it all at once. Is this a good idea?

No. Thyroid medication can expire like any other drug. This is especially true for natural thyroid medication, which may have an even shorter shelf life. Your pharmacist was trying to save you time, but unless you can be guaranteed the medication will not lose potency before you finish it, stick to filling your prescription every three months.

I've found a couple of online pharmacies that sell my thyroid medication for half the price. Is it okay to use them?

While some online pharmacies are reputable, watch out for sham pharmacies that sell expired or illegal medication. Beware of sites that do not require that you send in your doctor's prescription and do not guarantee their medications up until their expiration date. The best way to find a trustworthy online pharmacy is to ask your doctor for a recommendation. While it may cost you more money, it's a better idea to develop an ongoing relationship with an actual pharmacist, who is more likely to do a better job managing all your medications.

My pharmacist said I should try generic thyroid medication to save money, but my doctor won't prescribe it. Why not?

Some doctors believe that there are subtle differences between the generic and the brand-name thyroid medications, even though studies have shown that brand-name thyroid medication is not necessarily more effective than generic medication. Again, talk to your doctor about it. If you need to save money on your medicine, then your doctor needs to accommodate your situation.

Your coach
we all need someone to lean on

As you continue to build your support team, do not forget about the most important element: your personal advocate or coach. This is the one layperson you can trust to help you through difficult periods. Your coach can be your spouse, partner, relative, or good friend—basically, someone who will stand by your side and advocate for you when you encounter obstacles. Your coach should be open-minded, a good listener, and, above all, someone who respects your confidentiality.

Your coach should be willing to be a sounding board for the emotional ups and downs you are likely to face and also be willing to pitch in on practical matters, such as running errands when you are sick or watching your kids. It may seem like a lot to ask of someone, but a good coach gets a lot of pleasure out of helping others. And who knows? Someday you may be able to return the favor. A good coach or advocate is someone who:

◆ Stays informed about your illness, symptoms, and medications
◆ Keeps up-to-date about new treatments and advances
◆ Accompanies you on doctor's visits if you wish
◆ Is willing to deal with paperwork and make calls on your behalf
◆ Checks on you frequently, even if you claim to be fine

Some of the best advocates are those who have also suffered from the same condition as you or have loved ones struggling with it. If you do not know anyone willing to commit to being your coach, you might try joining a support group or online forum, where you will be able to get advice and support from others in the same boat.

Help was right around the corner

When I was diagnosed with thyroid cancer, my world caved in. As a lawyer and a single mother of two, I've been too busy to keep up ties with friends and family, so I felt I really had no one to turn to.

I decided to join an online cancer support group, and eventually I started corresponding with Adrienne, whose husband had recently passed away from thyroid lymphoma. It turned out that she lived only 15 minutes away. When we started meeting for coffee, I found her so helpful and supportive, and she knew everything about thyroid cancer. She even volunteered to come along with me on doctor's visits and asked tough questions I wouldn't have dared to ask. She really helped me through the tough times and listened to me when I got depressed about my illness.

When I went through treatment, she watched my kids and dropped by with a hot meal for us every Sunday. Then, when the doctor declared that my cancer was in remission, she organized a party for me—and boy, did we celebrate!

I've been cancer-free for two years now, and I have to say that, without Adrienne by my side, I don't know how I would have made it. I can't emphasize enough how important I think it is for anyone suffering from thyroid cancer to find someone like Adrienne to lean on. It made all the difference.

—Renee T., Chapel Hill, NC

Working with a psychotherapist
getting to the heart of the emotional symptoms

Here's how it can happen: Martha went undiagnosed with hypothyroidism for two years before finally getting correctly diagnosed. She is now on medication and is slowly returning to her old self. But during those two long years, there was much misery and her sense of self floundered. She lost all her self-confidence and her sense of well-being. Not surprising, her marriage suffered from her thyroid-induced depression.

Being of the old school, she found it hard to believe that her illness was partly to blame for her problems until her husband convinced her to visit a therapist trained in dealing with chronic illness. The therapist helped Martha understand that troubling psychological and sexual changes often go hand in hand with thyroid disorders. Sometimes these changes are caused by fluctuating hormone levels and sometimes they are the result of increased stress due to living with a chronic illness. The therapist helped Martha work through these issues, and her life is looking better.

The right therapist can make a huge difference when it comes to dealing with the psychological ramifications of living with a chronic illness. This is especially true of thyroid-disorder sufferers, who may not realize that their thyroid problem is a big part of their psychological problems. The same goes for your partner or loved ones, who may not realize that your thyroid disorder is causing them turmoil. They may pull away from you or react with anger or criticism without understanding the cause of their conflicted emotions. This is why adding a therapist to your support team at the first sign of trouble is such a good idea.

Before you visit a therapist, take a close look at your health journal and check for any major trends or changes in your emotional or mental state. Do your best to articulate these issues to the therapist, who will then be in a better position to work with you on these problems and help you repair any relationships negatively influenced by your illness.

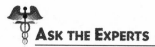

Ask the Experts

I have become increasingly anxious about my job. Is that normal?

That depends on what is going on at your office. However, one of the
hallmarks of hyperthyroidism is an increase in anxiety. In fact, some doctors find that the symptoms of an anxiety or panic attack can be
instances of hyperthyroidism.

**Ever since I was diagnosed with Graves' disease, I have been a lit-
tle bit on edge. I am trying to deal with it, but I don't want my loved
ones to feel that they have to treat me with kid gloves. What should
I do?**

It's normal after being diagnosed with any chronic illness to turn inward
and be more sensitive to the slings and arrows of everyday life. Just the
fact of being diagnosed with a chronic illness is a big stressor, more so
when the illness interferes with hormones that can affect your emotional
well-being. The solution is to give yourself time to adjust to your new situation. It's also a good idea to talk to a qualified therapist who can help
you sort out your new feelings.

**How do I find a psychotherapist who understands what life is like
with a chronic disease?**

Ask. Yes, it's that simple. When you are checking out therapists, ask
if they have had any experience with patients with a chronic illness and
the emotional repercussions.

Joining a support group
the great benefits of sharing your illness with others

Having a chronic illness can make you feel set apart from your family and friends. It can also feel like no one else can possibly understand what it's like to live with this day in and day out—not even your spouse or coach.

But you are wrong. There are several national organizations filled with people who share your situation. They draw strength from each other during their weekly support meetings or online through e-mail. They also play a very important role in treating thyroid disease by disseminating the latest research results, pushing for new legislation regarding medication and drug companies, and advocating for thyroid patients who may feel overlooked by their doctors.

Even more important, a thyroid support group can serve as a sounding board when you are having a particularly bad day—and they can help you put your suffering in perspective. Plus there will probably be at least one person in your group who has gone through experiences very similar to yours and may be able to provide valuable insight and emotional support.

Thyroid sufferers often say that joining a support group is the best thing they could have done. So why not give it a try? You will probably be surprised at how much strength you will be able to draw from others just like you.

To find a thyroid support group, start with the Thyroid Foundation of America, at **www.allthyroid.org,** which lists groups nationwide for people with various thyroid disorders. If you have thyroid cancer, try ThyCa (Thyroid Cancer Survivor's Organization and Conference), at **www.thyca.org**.

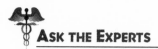

ASK THE EXPERTS

I don't really have time to join a support group. Are there online forums in which I can participate?

There are hundreds. The key is to find the one that's right for you. You will probably find the most help in a forum whose members are similar to you in terms of background (education, profession, age) and who are suffering from the same condition or symptoms, but this is not a hard-and-fast rule.

A few places to get started include **alt.support.thyroid** (a popular Usenet group), thyroid-related groups at Yahoo! and AOL, and Mary Shomon's Web site (**www.thyroid-info.org**), which hosts several forums specific to various thyroid concerns. The site also hosts a thyroid listserv to which you can subscribe. You can also try the Web sites of major thyroid organizations (see helpful resources on the next page).

When it comes to online forums, you need to be careful about sharing your medical information. Do not post highly confidential information in public forums, and if you want to share this information with another member, make sure you know and trust that person first.

Helpful resources

The Chronic Illness Workbook
by Patricia A. Fennell

The Thyroid Sourcebook
by M. Sara Rosenthal

*The Thyroid Solution: A
Revolutionary Mind-Body Program
That Will Help You*
by Ridha Arem, M.D.

Living Well with Hypothyroidism
by Mary J. Shomon

Thyroid Balance
by Glenn S. Rothfeld, M.D., M.Ac.,
and Deborah S. Romaine

*Thyroid Power: 10 Steps to Total
Health*
by Richard L. Shames, M.D., and
Karilee Halo Shames, R.N., Ph.D.

MAGIC Foundation
www.magicfoundation.org

**American Foundation of Thyroid
Patients**
www.thyroidfoundation.org

**National Graves' Disease
Foundation**
www.ngdf.org

Mary Shomon's Web site:
**www.thyroid-
info.com/topdrs/index.htm**

**American College for
Advancement in Medicine**
www.acam.org

The Role of Nutrition

Healthy eating
the principles of good nutrition

Having a chronic illness often causes people to reassess their eating habits. That can be a blessing, especially if your diet was not the greatest before you were diagnosed. Learning how to eat well can not only help you feel better but also give you back some control over your health. The question then is, what constitutes a healthy diet? If you follow the headlines, you may be confused over how to eat right. High protein or high carbohydrate? Low fat or high fat? Unlimited fruit or no fruit? Fortunately, the fundamentals of healthy eating are constant and quite simple to master. The right foods can do so much good. They can power your brain, fend off infections, and strengthen your muscles. By eating right you help shrink cholesterol, blood-sugar, and blood-pressure levels. And when your body has the food and nutrients it needs, you are less likely to be haunted by food cravings.

Keeping to a healthy diet is actually pretty straightforward. You need to eat a wide variety of fresh foods to ensure you get the proper amounts of nutrients and vitamins. And you need to watch your portion size. Proper serving size is most important to healthy eating. Many of us eat portions that are too big and supply too many calories. Portion sizes of packaged, take-out, and restaurant foods are often larger than necessary and filled with too many calories. It's no wonder that more and more of us are overweight! A registered dietitian (see pages 146–147) or weight-management program can offer you an individualized eating plan.

You also need to learn how your thyroid condition has affected your nutritional needs. If you are hypothyroid, you have probably suffered from bouts of constipation because your whole body was in low gear, including your digestive system. If you are hyperthyroid, you may have had spells of diarrhea that could have affected your nutritional needs.

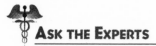

ASK THE EXPERTS

What is metabolism?

Metabolism is the total energy used by your body for all its processes. It has two components—**catabolism** (breaking down substances) and **anabolism** (storing energy). Hormones like thyroxine help regulate your metabolism by causing body processes to speed up or slow down. The hormone insulin influences how the body stores glucose from the breakdown of foods. Your "metabolic rate" is the number of calories your body burns in a 24-hour day to fuel basic body functions, along with digestion of food and physical activity.

I've heard salt is a problem when you have a thyroid condition. How much salt is too much?

Most Americans consume more than three teaspoons (8,000 milligrams or 8 grams) of salt each day. Most of that salt comes not from saltshakers but from processed foods. Check food labels. If you see the word *salt*, *soda*, or *sodium* high up in the ingredient list, then the product contains high amounts of sodium. Dietitians recommend limiting your daily salt intake to half a teaspoon (2,400 milligrams), regardless of whether you have a thyroid disorder or not.

Hypothyroid
slower metabolism means burning fewer calories

Hypothyroidism causes your body functions to slow down. (In other words, if your body were a car engine, your idle speed would be set too low.) Everything slows down. Even compounds in your blood like cholesterol are not processed normally.

Your weight You do not burn as many calories as you used to. If you have gained a lot of weight without good explanation, a slow thyroid may be the cause.

Digestive system Food takes longer to pass through your body. A slower-moving metabolism causes the intestines to remove a lot of fluid from food waste products. You become constipated because waste products need that fluid in order to be excreted normally. Gas and bloating are common side effects.

Cholesterol When you have hypothyroidism, your cholesterol and blood pressure may be higher than normal.

Energy level Hypothyroidism makes your engine slow down. Just as with cars, when your engine is not running fast enough, you cannot get very far very quickly. If you are also anemic, your blood cannot carry enough oxygen to your muscles to help them feel energized.

Diet and your treatment Once you start thyroid-hormone therapy and your metabolism returns to normal, your weight should drop. Studies show, however, that while weight does come off over the first few months of treatment, it gradually creeps back up. You need to make a conscious effort to eat healthfully, watch your portion size, and exercise.

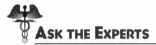

Ask the Experts

That first week or two after starting thyroid therapy, I felt very jittery. What should I do?

Check with your doctor. You could be getting too much thyroid hormone. Once you are on the right dosage, that jittery feeling should stop.

Will taking thyroid medication help my weight come off? Will I ever get back to my normal weight?

Your thyroid medication will help normalize your metabolism and increase your body's calorie burning. By itself, however, it will not take off all the extra pounds. The best strategy is to eat less and become more physically active. But don't starve yourself or overexercise—your body will think it's starving and will slow down its metabolism to prevent rapid weight loss.

What can I do for constipation?

Increase the amount of fiber in your diet by including plenty of fruits and vegetables, along with legumes (dried beans and peas) and foods made from whole grains. Starting your day with a bran cereal may also help. As you increase your fiber, remember to drink more water to help soften your stool and make it pass through your intestines more rapidly.

Hyperthyroid
fueling a faster metabolism

One of the consequences of having hyperthyroidism is that pounds simply melt away. Other symptoms include extreme restlessness, diarrhea, and exhaustion. In short, you are stuck in overdrive and your idle is too high.

Your weight Rapid, unintentional weight loss is one of the prime symptoms of hyperthyroidism. So is being hungrier than usual, again without a change in physical activity. You may find that you continue to lose weight although you are eating more.

Digestive system Your digestive system goes into overdrive from overstimulation by your body's abundance of thyroid hormones. Bowel movements are more frequent. Since your intestines have no time to extract the water from your waste products, expect to have bouts of diarrhea. Due to the increased loss of fluids in your bowel movements, you'll find yourself thirstier.

Cholesterol Hyperthyroidism does not cause major changes in blood levels of cholesterol and other compounds.

Energy level Hyperthyroidism can make you feel anxious and jittery, as if you drank too many cups of coffee. You may be restless and have difficulty sitting still or sleeping. The flip side—you also feel worn out from your body's running at such a fast speed. Coffee, tea, and caffeinated soft drinks can prevent you from sleeping properly, especially if you drink them in the late afternoon or evening.

Diet and your treatment

The goal of your treatment is to return your thyroid-hormone levels to normal. With that, your metabolism slows, meaning that you need fewer calories. You are likely to feel less hungry, so listen to your stomach and cut back on your eating. Otherwise, you will gain weight.

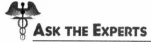
Should I avoid certain foods when I have diarrhea?

For starters, avoid any foods that gave you loose bowel movements or diarrhea before you developed thyroid disease. You may want to keep a diary to record what you eat and when you have diarrhea to help pinpoint problem foods. Here are some common culprits: Milk and many dairy products are broken down by an enzyme called lactase. Many healthy adults do not produce enough lactase and get diarrhea from milk. Faster than normal intestinal movement makes absorbing fat difficult, so high-fat foods may cause diarrhea.

FIRST PERSON INSIGHTS

The wrong way to lose weight

I noticed the weight loss first. How could I not? After years of being overweight, it seemed like a miracle to be shedding pounds and still be able to eat normally. After a time, other symptoms started to develop. I was very restless and extremely irritable. I also had a terrible case of diarrhea. But still the pounds kept coming off and people were complimenting me on my new slim shape. When I went for my checkup, my doctor was concerned about my weight loss and tested me for a thyroid disorder. He told me I had Graves' disease and prescribed medication to calm down my thyroid gland. After a month, the weight started coming back on. It was as if I was going back to my old self. I was feeling fine, and I decided to stop taking the medicine so I wouldn't get fat again. But after a while, all the old hyperthyroid symptoms came back. When I went for my three-month checkup, my doctor was dumfounded at the results, until I told him I had stopped taking the pills. He very quietly explained that my health was more important than my figure. Being hyperthyroid can cause a number of serious health problems. I needed to take my medicine and watch what I ate. I did as the doctor ordered. I gained a few pounds back, but I am sticking to my diet now.

—Gail S., Sandy Hook, VA

Hashimoto's disease and food
Food can help strengthen your immunity

When your immune system becomes too aggressive and attacks your body's own cells or organs, you develop what is called an autoimmune disease. With Hashimoto's disease, the thyroid gland comes under attack by the body's own white blood cells and antibodies, leading to inflammation. Diet planning is a challenge since metabolism is normal, or even too fast, in the early stages of Hashimoto's, but right after treatment, hypothyroidism and its lethargic effects come on. The result is a slowed metabolism and weight gain. In due time, your metabolism will return to normal as your body learns to adjust to its hormone treatment.

Not surprisingly, this hormonal roller coaster can wreak havoc on your metabolism. The good news is that your metabolism should return to normal once you are on replacement thyroid hormone. Meanwhile, you may be concerned about how to deal with the excess weight you most likely gained during your bout with Hashimoto's disease. You have several options:

♦ **Follow the fundamentals of healthy eating** detailed on pages 144–145, taking care to eat less food than you have been eating. Increase your physical activity to burn additional calories.

♦ **Join a group** Weight Watchers and others offer weekly classes, guidance, and group support to help people lose weight and keep the pounds off. Online weight-loss support groups are also available.

♦ **Work with a dietitian** (see pages 146–147). A registered dietitian will tailor a weight-loss program to your food likes and dislikes, as well as your medical needs. Some dietitians offer online counseling in place of office visits.

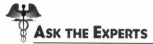

ASK THE EXPERTS

I am so upset about my weight gain, I am ready to try just about anything. I heard about a weight-loss program that guarantees that I'll lose five pounds a week. Is that healthy?

Be wary of programs that promise dramatic weight loss. Weight loss should be slow and steady—no more than one to two pounds a week. A goal of slow weight loss gives you more time to change your eating habits, and weight lost slowly may be easier to keep off. Much of the weight lost quickly is water weight, which is quick to come back. Steer clear of programs that blame weight gain on particular types of foods and tell you to eliminate entire food groups—for example, grain products. Grain foods supply fiber and other important nutrients that are tough to replace with other foods.

Dieter, beware

Avoid any diets or weight-loss products that:

♦ Pronounce certain foods as good or bad.
("Pineapple will burn the fat.")

♦ Use someone else's results to predict yours.
("Jim here lost 40 pounds in 60 days. You can, too!")

♦ Promise quick and effortless results.
("Just one pill a day and you will lose weight.")

♦ Are based on studies that have not been reviewed by bona fide nutritional groups.
("This product has been reviewed by the Council of Herbologists and found to be safe and effective.")

Graves' disease and food

food can help strengthen your immunity

Like Hashimoto's disease, Graves' disease is an autoimmune disorder. But here your metabolism is so revved up, you lose weight and feel jittery and restless. The other main symptom of Graves' disease is diarrhea. Excess thyroid hormone speeds up every process in your body, including how quickly your intestines contract to push food through. This overstimulation of your intestinal tract can lead to diarrhea because your intestines do not have enough time to absorb fluid and nutrients from the foods you eat. Diarrhea means that you are losing fluid, along with nutrients like fat and minerals. Severe loss of nutrients can lead to malnutrition, a withering away of the inner surface of your intestine, and a worsening of your diarrhea. Once you begin hyperthyroid treatment, your diarrhea should abate. Also, in the early stages of treatment, you may lose weight without trying because your metabolism is faster than normal. As your Graves' disease is treated and your thyroid-hormone production drops, your metabolism will slow, reducing your calorie needs.

In the meantime, you might want to consider:

◆ **Cutting back on dairy** Lactose, the sugar in milk, is difficult to digest for many adults and especially for people with unhealthy intestines. Undigested lactose causes extra fluid to be secreted into the intestine and can cause diarrhea.

◆ **A low-fat diet** Fat is hard to digest and absorb if your intestine is not healthy; the intestinal surface produces enzymes that help break fat into smaller particles that can be absorbed. Without enough enzymes, your body does not digest fat completely, leading to loose stools.

Calcium caution

Hyperthyroidism not only speeds up your metabolism, it also speeds up metabolism in your bones, causing them to lose too much calcium. Excess loss of calcium from your bones can lead to osteoporosis (porous bones). The result is brittle bones that break easily. Treatment that returns your thyroid-hormone levels to normal will lessen your risk of developing hyperthyroid-induced osteoporosis.

Getting enough calcium—1,000 milligrams (mg) daily through age 50 and 1,200 mg if you're 51 or older—helps maintain bone strength. Include two to three servings of milk, yogurt, or other high-calcium foods in your daily diet. Regular, weight-bearing exercise like walking, jogging, or using an elliptical machine at the gym boosts bone strength. Vitamin D, found primarily in fortified milk, yogurt, and breakfast cereal, boosts calcium absorption. Your body also makes vitamin D from sunlight. Talk to your doctor about whether a vitamin D supplement is advisable. Also talk to your doctor about taking a calcium supplement, as this can lower levels of Synthroid in the blood. To avoid this negative interaction, take the calcium four hours before or after you take your Synthroid.

Graves' and Celiac Disease

There is a correlation between Graves' and Celiac disease—in which the body develops an intolerance to the protein gluten (found in wheat). Symptoms include bloating, gas, and diarrhea, especially shortly after eating wheat products. Only a small percentage of the population has Celiac disease, but it is more prevalent in people with an autoimmune thyroid disease like Graves' or Hashimoto's. Talk to your doctor if you suspect that you may be having reactions to foods made with wheat.

Boosting your immune system
food can help strengthen your immunity

Your immune system helps protect your body from illness. When your immune system malfunctions—it is either not active enough or too active—you get sick. Eating certain foods does not guarantee that your immune system will stay healthy, but a healthy diet can help your immune system work at its best.

Vitamins and minerals

Certain vitamins and minerals in the foods you eat play an important role in the health of your immune system.

Vitamins A and C, along with the minerals zinc, selenium, and iron, are known to help keep the immune system working at its best. Fruits and vegetables are a top source of vitamins A and C, while meats are particularly high in zinc and iron. Whole grains supply selenium.

Vitamin E, found in nuts and vegetable oils, may protect immune cells from damage and help the body maintain its normal immunity, particularly in older adults.

Vitamin D and calcium may help lessen the chances of developing certain autoimmune diseases, according to preliminary studies on animals. You can meet your daily vitamin D recommendations by including milk, vitamin-D fortified yogurt, fortified breakfast cereal, and other foods and beverages fortified with vitamin D in your diet, as well as by being exposed to sunlight (your body makes vitamin D from sunlight). Don't overdo it—vitamin D is stored in the body, and too much can be dangerous—and speak to your doctor or dietitian if you have questions about whether you are getting enough.

Focus on fish

Higher-fat fish like salmon, sardines, tuna, sea bass, herring, and mackerel have an abundance of a certain type of fat, called omega-3, that appears to help the immune system in healthy people as well as people with certain autoimmune diseases. The body converts omega-3 fatty acids into hormone-like compounds needed for a normal immune response. You can get your omega-3's by following the recommendations of the American Heart Association, the American Dietetic Association, and others to eat fish at least twice weekly, and include higher-fat fish when possible. Note: Omega-3 also helps lower your risk of heart disease. Some people prefer to take fish-oil supplements that supply omega-3's; discuss the pros and cons of these supplements with your doctor or dietitian.

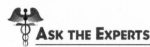

ASK THE EXPERTS

Should I avoid shellfish if I have a thyroid condition?

No. You need only refrain from eating shellfish if you are having a radioactive iodine uptake scan. Otherwise, eat as much as you want. There is not enough iodine in shellfish to have any impact on your thyroid.

Portion control
the principles of good nutrition

The key to healthy eating lies in portion control. The U.S. Department of Agriculture's Food Guide Pyramid recommends a range of servings per day from each food group. If you are trying to lose weight, start with the lowest number of servings recommended.

Include grain foods like bread, cereal, pasta, and rice

Why? Your body needs these grain foods for their carbohydrates, the body's top energy source. Grains also supply important minerals and B vitamins. To get enough fiber, choose whole grains whenever possible; for example, a whole-grain cereal at breakfast and a whole-wheat bread sandwich for lunch.

Eat: 6 to 11 servings daily (each meal may have more than one serving)

Food	Serving Size	Common Measure
Bagel	1/2 small	1/2 packaged English muffin
Bread, toast	1 slice	Slice from standard loaf
Breakfast cereal	1 cup	Standard teacup
Pasta or rice	1/2 cup cooked	Cupped palm

Include fruits and vegetables

Why? Fruits and vegetables dish up vitamins A and C, fiber, and a slew of natural compounds that are good for overall health. They are also filling and relatively low in calories.

Eat: 2 to 4 servings of fruit; 3 to 5 servings (or more) of vegetables daily

Food	Serving Size	Common Measure
Fruit	1 medium	Baseball
Fruit juice	6 fluid ounces	Juice glass
Vegetables	1/2 cup	Bulb portion of lightbulb

Include dairy products

Why? Dairy products like milk and yogurt supply calcium, the mineral necessary to build strong bones. Calcium is particularly important for those at high risk of osteoporosis—older women and people with hyperthyroidism. Cheese also supplies calcium but is higher in fat and calories. To control calories, choose reduced-fat cheese, along with low-fat or nonfat milk and yogurt. Try calcium-fortified juice or soy milk if you do not use dairy products.

Eat: 2 to 3 servings daily

Food	Serving Size	Common Measure
Cheese	1 ounce	2 dominos
Milk, yogurt	1 cup	Standard yogurt container
Fortified juice	1 cup	Standard yogurt container

Include a variety of proteins

Why? Meat, poultry, fish, beans, eggs, and nuts all supply protein, the nutrient your body needs to build and repair muscle and tissue. Each also offers its own unique benefits; for example, meat is high in iron and zinc, fish supplies omega-3 fatty acids, and beans have fiber. The Food Guide Pyramid recommends relatively small portions.

Eat: 2 servings daily

Food	Serving Size	Common Measure
Beans (kidney, pinto, etc.)	1/2 cup (replaces 1 ounce meat)	Bulb portion of lightbulb
Eggs	1 (replaces 1 ounce meat)	Large egg
Meat, chicken, fish	3 ounces	Palm of a woman's hand
Peanut butter	2 tablespoons	1 walnut

Finding nutritional help
diet professionals can make all the difference

Try as you might, it can be hard to find a diet that works for you. It can be even harder to turn that diet into a lifelong pattern of healthy eating. This is especially true if you have to factor in thyroid-hormonal swings. If your weight loss plan is not going as well as you want, don't be discouraged. Instead seek out some professional support. The best person to hire is a registered dietitian. She can teach you about the basics of healthful eating and about making specific changes in your diet for thyroid disorders (as well as other health issues you may have).

At your first appointment, a registered dietitian will review your medical history, ask you questions about your current diet, and plan changes to your eating habits that are appropriate for your illness. Follow-up appointments will review your progress and adjust your diet as needed for your condition. Consultation with a registered dietitian (or R.D.) for medical purposes is covered by some, but not all, insurance plans, so check with your insurance company regarding coverage. Also be sure to ask your doctor for the names of dietitians she recommends for patients with thyroid conditions.

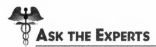

Ask the Experts

What is the difference between a nutritionist and a registered dietitian?

A nutritionist has studied nutrition and often has received a master's degree. Registered dietitians are health professionals who have completed an accredited education and training program and have passed a national credentialing exam. Many registered dietitians also have master's degrees in nutrition.

How do I find a dietitian?

You can find a dietitian on your own through the Yellow Pages or by contacting the American Dietetic Association at 800 877-1600, ext. 5000, or at **www.eatright.org**. Begin by asking for names of dietitians in your area, or ask your insurance carrier for the names of approved providers.

Helpful resources

Thyroid Disease: The Facts
(Oxford Medical Publications)
by R.I.S. Bayliss and
W.M.G. Tunbridge
Offers practical advice about the
thyroid gland and its disorders.

*American Dietetic Association
Complete Food and Nutrition Guide
(2nd Edition)*
by Roberta Larson Duyff, M.S.,
R.D., C.F.C.S., American
Dietetic Association
Sound advice on healthful eating,
including chapters on nutrition and
health conditions and on dietary
supplements.

Dieting for Dummies
by Jane Kirby, American
Dietetic Association
Practical, easy-to-understand
advice on weight management and
weight loss.

American Dietetic Association
Tel: 800 877-1600
www.eatright.org
Offers nutrition information,
including consumer tips, fact sheets,
FAQs, resources, and referrals to
dietitians.

American Foundation of Thyroid
Patients
Tel: 281 855-6608
www.thyroidfoundation.org
An organization that was founded
by thyroid patients and is governed
and directed solely for the purpose
of education and support of thyroid
patients.

Choosing a Safe and Successful
Weight-Loss Program
www.niddk.nih.gov/health/
nutrit/pubs/choose.htm
Government guidelines on evaluating and selecting a weight-loss program.

Food and Nutrition Information
Center
www.nal.usda.gov/fnic/pubs/bibs
/topics/weight/consumer.html
Resources compiled by the U.S.
Department of Agriculture, includ-
ing a Weight Control and Obesity
Resource List for Consumers.

On Stress and Comfort

What is stress?

it's not just a built-in survival mechanism

The alarm rings. You wake up startled and race for the shower. Then it's coffee and the morning rush. You work through lunch, then it's phone calls and e-mails. On and on it goes, until you come home staggering and exhausted. Welcome to the world of stress. Not surprisingly, *stress* has become the watchword of the millennium.

It seems that stress can cause certain illnesses as well as worsen your symptoms once you become ill. How can stress cause illness as well as worsen its symptoms? The answer lies in the very complex nature of stress—or, rather, our complex reaction to it. While scientists have learned a great deal more about the nature of stress in the past few years, they are still baffled by it. One of the most puzzling aspects of stress is that its effect on our bodies is based on how we perceive stressful situations. Some stress can help us perform at our peak abilities, such as competing in a race. Other stress can be debilitating, such as an unwanted divorce or a job loss. It's all in the eye of the beholder.

A perceived short-term threat

When it comes to short-term stress, there is a fairly universal understanding of it. In fact, surviving sudden threats is so critical to our survival that our bodies are designed to either fight or flee the threat. Here's how our bodies handle it: When a threat is perceived, the brain's hypothalamus sends out an alarm to the sympathetic nervous system to release adrenaline into the bloodstream. This increases your heart rate and blood pressure so you can run or fight. It also drains blood from the brain. That means the brain is getting less oxygen, and this in turn makes rational thinking a lot harder. (Ever wonder why people sometimes freeze in the face of danger or do something really irrational? It's because they get so light-headed they literally cannot think of what to do.)

Next the brain signals the adrenal glands to release epinephrine and nor-epinephrine hormones. These hormones increase the glucose levels in the blood so that muscles can effectively respond. This is why some people can perform incredible feats of strength in a crisis. Note: The perceived threat is always in the eye of the beholder. The stress response will occur whether the threat is real or imagined; (That is the reason your heart races during a scary movie.)

Once the threat has passed, the brain issues an "all-clear" signal. Neurons, special cells in the brain, send out signals to the major organs to return to normal. This allows the digestive system to go back to the business of digesting food, and the heart returns to a calmer beat. Essentially, the body is told to relax—the threat is over. If the threat lasted for a few minutes, ideally it will take a few minutes for the body to return to normal.

Women and Stress

Women react differently to stress

For the past 50 years, stress research has been done on male animals. It was from their response to various stressors that researchers came up with the catchphrase "fight or flight." That changed in 1998 when researcher Shelley E. Taylor decided to study the stress response in female animals. Dr. Taylor found that females responded differently to nonlife-threatening stress, particularly if they were tending young offspring. These animals did not become nearly as alarmed as their male counterparts. In fact, their reaction was to tend to their young and to seek comfort in other females. Dr. Taylor went on to test her theory on men and women and found that in general men tend to isolate themselves when they feel stressed, while women confide their problems to each other. As Dr. Taylor describes it in her book, *The Tending Instinct,* women "tend and befriend."

Chronic stress

be alert to coping patterns

What happens when a perceived threat lingers for days or weeks? Long-term negative stressors, such as a messy divorce, becoming ill, or being laid off from work, may go on for months. This means the all-clear signal is never given by the brain, and the body never gets a chance to return to equilibrium. It's as if the body is in a constant state of alert. Over time, this can take a physical toll on the body, especially if these stressors are perceived to be negative threats. Again, perception is key. This is why some people thrive on such stressors as deadlines for a project they are passionate about, and why others who don't feel emotionally involved or in control of their work feel "stressed out."

Long-term negative stress can lead to bouts of anxiety, aggression, and depression. Some scientists believe that chronic stress has a harmful effect on the immune system and the endocrine system, making people more vulnerable to illness and infections. Whether you have an illness or not, when it comes to chronic stress, you need to try to improve your coping skills.

So how do you cope with long-term stress? For starters, look at how you have coped in the past. Did you isolate yourself from friends and family? Did you seek out comfort foods? sleep a lot? fall into bad habits, such as overeating or drinking? Try to see if there is a pattern to how you coped. It's also a good idea to recall how your parents or other significant caregivers handled negative stressors. You may have internalized their coping responses and not realized it.

Negative coping responses

There are several negative coping responses that we have all used at one time or another when dealing with long-term stress. Here is a round-up:

- **Deny the problem** This is a common response for many people—they simply ignore the problem. Often, to help take their minds off the problem, they throw themselves into their work or social life.

- **Dwell on your problems** Again, this is usually a learned response. Did your parents or caregivers fret excessively over your health as you were growing up? Or did they ignore your health completely? If they did either of these extremes, you may find yourself obsessing about your health. If these thoughts become chronic, you should see a therapist who can help you break the pattern of obsessive rumination.

- **Procrastinate decision making** Instead of thinking through the problems at hand, you endlessly analyze the situation and talk about the same problems and solutions over and over again with friends and family.

- **Seek thrills** You look for excitement or experiences to distract you from your problems.

- **Get angry and vent to others** This is known as displaced aggression. You take out your anger at being ill on others and overreact to their responses.

- **Withdraw** You physically or emotionally withdraw from others. People under chronic stress will often cope by sleeping excessively or simply by disengaging from the world.

- **Overindulge** Food is used as a drug to mask fears as well as boredom. Too much alcohol is another negative way to cope with all the problems of chronic stress.

Smart coping strategies
find positive ways to cope with chronic problems

Dealing with chronic stress can tap your coping reserves. Your old favorite coping standbys may work, but not for the long haul. The challenge of coping with long-term stress is understanding how to live with it. This calls for a new way of looking at your health and looking at illness. Since there is no cure for stress, the goal becomes the reduction of your discomfort. That means really listening to your symptoms and addressing them. Your goal is simply to improve your quality of life. Here are some coping tips to help you on your way.

Focus on favorite activities If certain hobbies or activities, such as cooking a gourmet meal, going to the movies, playing sports, or reading mystery stories, were your means of getting away from it all in the past, chances are they still will be. Moreover, they now can be a retreat from your new stress.

Get organized Time management becomes a tool you can really use when you have a chronic illness. Your time and energy are now precious commodities that should not be wasted. Learn how to separate out those things you really need to do from those you can spread out over time or delegate to others.

Develop healthy habits Ironically, people often become healthier once they have been diagnosed with a chronic illness. This may be because they suddenly stop taking their health for granted and turn negative habits into healthy ones, such as maintaining a good diet (see pages 131–148) or quitting smoking.

Make attitude adjustments Life with chronic stress can make the world a dour place. Put some humor back in your life. Rent funny movies and read humorous books and magazines.

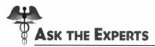
I have to travel for work. How can I cut down on stress while I'm on the road?

Traveling is a big stressor, doubly so if you have to manage a chronic illness while you are on the road. It's smart to be proactive and plan ahead as much as possible. For starters, create a small health file with the phone numbers and contact information for all the people on your support team (see pages 110–130). Make sure to bring extra medication, just in case. Next, don't just pack for your trip. Bring a bit of home with you. Include a pair of comfortable jeans or a favorite shawl. Some people who hate to travel bring photos of their family and put them in their hotel room. Don't forget to bring a novel, computer games, knitting, or whatever else you like to do to relax.

FIRST PERSON INSIGHTS

Too close for comfort

For me, the hardest part of being diagnosed with full-blown Hashimoto's disease was talking about it. The minute I told this one close friend, she went overboard. She called to check on me every day and sent me cards and notes. For a while it was kind of sweet, then it got a bit out of hand. She wanted to know everything about my treatment. After a time, I dreaded talking to her and stopped taking her calls. Finally, I explained that her attention was making me nervous and I needed to focus on getting well. She apologized and backed off. I am glad I set some boundaries and took control of the situation. We are still friends, but I am mindful of what I talk about.

—Sarah M., Miami , FL

Learning to relax
beat chronic stress at its own game

Our bodies are brilliantly designed to handle stress. They are also designed to handle relaxation. In fact, the stress response and the relaxation response are both hardwired into our brains. Doctors are just now beginning to understand the power of relaxation upon the body—both to rejuvenate and to heal.

Think back to a time when you felt truly relaxed. What was going on? You were probably in a quiet, comfortable space where you had no pressures to do anything but sit back and enjoy the day. You felt peaceful and at one with the world. For most people, that is the definition of a vacation. Here's the news flash: To be healthy, your body needs a little vacation every day. How do you achieve that? Here are some tips:

Quiet time Carve out 10 minutes of the day simply to quietly "be." Meditation practices are very helpful in teaching people how to still their minds and relax. See pages 104–105 for more on this.

Deep breathing When you are stressed, your breathing becomes shortened, so much so that you can hyperventilate when faced with acute stress. Counter this natural instinct by purposefully taking four deep breaths every time you feel stressed. Breathe in through your nose, hold the breath for five seconds, and then release the air through your mouth for five seconds.

Exercise Chronic muscle tension is part and parcel of a chronic stress response. Counteract it by taking a walk or playing a round of tennis. Your goal is to keep your body limber and to keep it moving. For a more relaxing exercise, consider taking a class in yoga or tai chi (see pages 106–107 for more information). Note: Massage is a great way to help rid your muscles of stress-related tension (see pages 100–101).

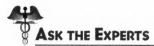

ASK THE EXPERTS

I have been stressed out for so long, I don't think anything will help.

If you have been enduring chronic stressors for a long period of time, trying to relax overnight is not going to work. In fact, it will just make you more stressed. You need to retrain your body on how to feel and behave while relaxed. Consider taking a short-term workshop to help you learn how to relax. Your doctor can refer you to a stress clinic or a stress specialist. You can take courses in stress management. The American Management Association offers two-day workshops on managing stress; call 800-262-9699. Or try your local YMCA or YMHA—they usually offer stress-management classes.

I heard that writing about stressful events can help you get over them. Is that true?

Yes, there are some studies that show that writing about stressful issues or traumatic experiences can help improve the immune system. Use your health journal (see pages 14–15) to write about your concerns.

Talking about it
learn how to talk about your needs

For some people, talking about what stresses them is torturous. For others, it's their favorite pastime. Where do you stand in the equation? If your job or your thyroid condition is causing you concern, you really should share this with close friends and family. If you don't talk about it, you run the risk of isolating yourself from your friends and family. If you find it uncomfortable to talk about your problems, here are a few tips to make it easier:

1. Pick the time and place to talk. You need to set a time and place that is comfortable for you. Don't get backed into talking about your illness when you are not ready. You need to feel in control of the conversation, and picking the time and place will help you feel in charge.

2. Rehearse what you want to say out loud in front of a mirror before you actually talk to your spouse or friends. Saying the words out loud for yourself can help take the sting out of them.

3. Set the terms and limits of the information you want to share. You are the one in charge here, so do not let anyone take over the conversation and ask you invasive questions. Simply call a halt to the questions and say you don't feel comfortable answering them right now. Also, set the terms of your information. If you don't want this information shared with others, then say so. Here's an example: "Joanie, I have been wanting to talk to you about something important that is going on in my life right now. At this time, I don't want this information shared with others. Is that agreeable to you?"

4. Think about whom you are telling and what you want that person to say to your news. If you want emotional support, say so. Don't expect hugs from everyone. Emotional support may be easy to get from empathetic types, but unlikely from those who pride themselves solely on their intellect and reasoning abilities.

Learn how not to talk about it

It's only natural to assume that because something interests you intensely, then it must also interest everyone else. And if that something is as all-important as your thyroid disorder, your family and close friends will want to know every detail, and even casual acquaintances will be fascinated by the dramatic story line. Wrong. Remind yourself every day that a good conversationalist is first of all a good listener. Ask questions about things that interest other people, and listen—really listen—to the answers. Have things to talk about besides you and your health concerns.

Five Rules for Talking about Your Illness

1. "How are you?" is a salutation, not a request for medical news. Just because you have a chronic illness, there is no reason to change your usual response. Wait until someone asks specifically about your illness before telling them about it.

2. Fit the answer to your audience. Have a short version and a long version ready. Your spouse may want to hear all about your doctor's visit, but your colleagues want only a summary version.

3. Watch for eyes glazing over. Someone has asked about your illness and seems really interested. So you launch into the long version. Watch for signs that you may have misjudged. Does he fidget? glance around? If you pause or ask a question, is there a slight delay before you have his attention again?

4. After three minutes, change the subject. Even the most loving friend may not be able to take in every detail of an extended medical report. Give them a break. Anyone who is really interested will return to the subject.

5. Use humor. Have a couple of jokes handy to break up your monologue, or provide an exit line.

Your partner's concerns
how thyroid troubles can impact relationships

Having any illness usually calls for couples to reassess their partnership. If it's a temporary illness, then it's usually a question of juggling practical matters, such as "Who will pick up the kids while I am at the doctor?" But when symptoms are no longer signs of a temporary illness but the manifestation of a chronic illness, a bigger reassessment is needed. Couples need to look at each other's roles and responsibilities in the relationship. You need to state which changes you need to make. This may mean reassigning roles, whether cleaning duties or paying the bills. Often, couples fall into the trap where one becomes the dominant caregiver and the other becomes the professional patient. Try to avoid that dynamic, because it usually leads to resentment on both sides. It's a good idea to have your spouse come along with you on a doctor's visit so he or she can see firsthand what it's like to be a patient.

Money may become an issue if you do not have adequate health insurance or need to cut back on work (see pages 162–163). Illness can also affect your sex life. Thyroid disorders often result in weight gain and fatigue—symptoms that can have a big impact on your sex life. Talk about your concerns and listen to your partner. The important thing is to keep the lines of communication open, and not shut down. It's a good idea for couples to see a therapist to work through some of these issues. A good therapist, knowledgeable about the effects of chronic disease on sexuality, may be able to help you work through these issues. To find a therapist for your particular concern, start at the American Association of Sex Educators, Counselors, and Therapists (**www.aasect.org**). Also check with the larger thyroid-support foundations to see if they host any spouse-support groups. If not, you can always start your own or start an online spouses' forum. At **www.thyroid.about.com**, you can find some excellent tips for starting your own support group.

Telling the children

How to talk about your chronic illness

How do you tell your children that you have a chronic illness? It depends on how much this illness has affected your health. In the case of thyroid disorders, it can take quite a while for symptoms to abate. If those symptoms cause significant changes in your parenting style, then you need to tell your children how your illness has affected you.

If you have young children, pick a quiet time and place to talk about it. Ask your partner to be present at this meeting. Use easy-to-understand language. Be as specific as you can: "Remember when Mommy couldn't take you to the swimming pool because she was too tired? Well, the reason is Mommy has an illness, but she is getting better. But until she is all better, we need to work out together how to do some things. Let's ask Aunt Sandy or Uncle Mike to take you to the swimming pool. How does that sound?"

Older children will want to know more details. Again, be specific, and use concrete examples of how the illness has affected you. Rehearse what you want to say. The most important thing is to assure your children that you are not in any danger. Reassure them that you and they will be just fine.

Managing the inconveniences
dealing with the hard issues

There are a number of inconveniences involved when you have a chronic illness. They usually come down to two things: time and money. If your thyroid symptoms are still troubling you, then you are bound to find yourself canceling social engagements or perhaps rearranging your work schedule. Then, of course, there are the myriad doctor's appointments you need to factor into your already busy schedule. This is not fun.

Next comes a real stressor for those with any chronic illness: paying for it. If you do not have health insurance, having a chronic illness can be very costly. You will need to find low-cost clinics that can help you manage your illness. And since most thyroid disorders require lifelong medication, you will need to find prescription drugs that you can afford. If you are over 65, you can apply for Medicaid. For those with health insurance, one of the most stressful aspects of your illness will be managing the multiple forms you will need to present to get coverage for your health care.

Finally, having a chronic illness can sometimes influence your work life. You may find that you need to cut back on your hours or reduce your schedule to part-time. Some may find that they have to stop working altogether until they are back on the road to health. The good news is that the American Disabilities Act can protect you from being fired because of your illness. Employers who have more than 50 people working for them are required by law to try and make some kind of accommodation with you once you have been diagnosed with a chronic illness or disability.

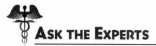

ASK THE EXPERTS

I am in between jobs right now and don't have any health insurance. How do I find inexpensive health insurance that will cover my preexisting thyroid condition?

You want to consider health-insurance coverage that is based on membership instead of employment. Consider joining a trade or professional organization that has its own health insurance. For example, if you are a graphic artist, you can join the American Institute of Graphic Artists. It offers an insurance plan to its members, and once you join you may become eligible for it.

I have had to miss a couple of days of work to undergo more thyroid tests. Should I tell my boss about my thyroid condition?

This is totally up to you. It's not necessary to "go public" about your health to your employer unless your performance at work is suffering because of it. Only you can know that. Everyone gets sick from time to time. You should not be made to feel guilty about taking your allotted sick days. If you find you need more time off because of your thyroid condition, then yes, you do need to explain your situation to your boss. See pages 158–159 on how to talk about having a chronic illness. Thanks to the American Disabilities Act, once you inform your employer about your health condition, you cannot be fired because of it. You need to work with your boss to accommodate both your health needs and the needs of the business.

Helpful resources

*Difficult Conversations: How to
Discuss What Matters Most*
by Douglas Stone, Sheila Heen,
and Bruce Patton

The Chronic Illness Workbook
by Patricia Fennell

*Insurance Solutions:
A Workbook for People with a
Chronic Disease or Disability*
by Laura D. Cooper

Recrafting a Life
by Charlie Johnson and
Denise Webster

The Tending Instinct
by Shelley E. Taylor

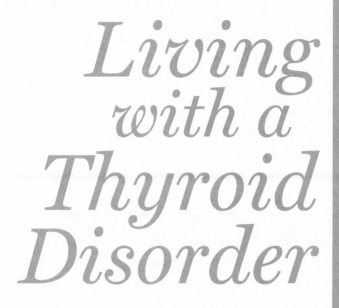

CHAPTER 10

Living with a Thyroid Disorder

Life with a thyroid disorder
it can be a rocky road

In your not too distant past, whenever you got sick you went to the doctor, probably got a prescription, felt better, and went on with your life. Depending on your situation, that could have changed the day you received the diagnosis that you had a thyroid disorder. Whether it is Hashimoto's or Graves' disease, or simply a low-functioning thyroid, you have found yourself up against something for which medical science has yet to find a cure. The good news, of course, is that thyroid disorders are rarely life-threatening. Moreover, the treatment for most thyroid disorders is very easy—a pill every day.

Most people do fine with their daily hormone therapy. Their symptoms abate, and they get on with their lives. Remembering to take the medicine every single day at the same time can prove to be annoying occasionally, but it is a small price to pay to feel like yourself again.

But some people aren't so lucky. They still suffer from symptoms, despite their treatment. There are several reasons for this. The problem may be:

- **The wrong thyroid medication** There are several generic and brand-name thyroid medications to choose from. There are synthetic and natural thyroid hormones to consider, too. Some people feel better on the synthetic hormones, while some prefer the natural. Some find the generic drugs to be just fine; others do well only with the brand names.

- **The wrong dosage** Along with finding the right type of drug, having the right amount is key. Too little, and symptoms return; too much, and other symptoms ensue.

- **Body changes** Big physical changes, such as pregnancy and childbirth, an injury, or an illness, can affect your thyroid and require adjustments to your medication. Aging and menopause will also call for adjustments to thyroid medication.

It can be very frustrating to try different drugs and dosages, waiting and hoping to see if they work. And it can be very hard to start to feel symptoms again for no apparent reason other than the fact that you have turned 60. Not surprisingly, you can sometimes feel like a walking chemistry experiment. This experiment becomes all the harder because you are the one who is required to report your symptoms to your doctor, who may become as frustrated as you if you show no improvement.

Learning how to keep track of your symptoms is key. A lot of people have trouble with this. But ignoring your symptoms can be downright dangerous. There is a fine line between paying attention to your symptoms and dwelling on them. This is one reason your doctor will ask if your symptoms are interfering with your daily life. Keeping a health journal can help you track your feelings and symptoms (see pages 14–15). Make it your special place to record your feelings, both physical and emotional. Use your journal to help chart a road map to health.

Stages of adjustment
from the old you to the new you

Attitude is everything. As doctors start to realize the healing power of the mind, they are paying more attention to helping their patients psychologically cope with chronic illness. Accepting that you have a medical condition is the first step. This is not as easy as it sounds. Some researchers believe that coping with a chronic illness, even one as minor as a thyroid disorder, entails grieving over one's lost health. There is a range of emotions to go through, which are similar to those explained by Elisabeth Kübler-Ross in her groundbreaking book *On Death and Dying*. Those stages of grief are anger, denial, bargaining, depression, and acceptance. There is no prescribed order or set time to these stages.

Denial

Once you get that diagnosis, you realize that your thyroid disorder is something you will always need to be aware of. You can no longer take your health for granted, even though this illness is treatable. That can be a bitter pill for some people to swallow, especially young people who have never had a health issue. Not surprisingly, they choose to ignore it. Some even go so far as not to take their medication. What's the reason for this? For most people, it's fear and shame. Lingering symptoms of thyroid disease can be very frightening. Some people feel ashamed that their body has betrayed them. Add to that a loss of personal power, which is an important contributor to self-esteem. It's no wonder that they may simply deny the problem.

What to do Be kind to yourself. Coping with all these issues can be overwhelming. Every person who has experienced strange medical symptoms is frightened. So take some time and try to think through the situation. What would you tell a friend who was experiencing strange physical symptoms? Probably the same thing your family and friends are telling you. You are not at fault. Go back to your doctor and work on finding a treatment plan that works for you.

Anger, Depression, and Bargaining

You may find yourself saying something like this: "I see my doctor for thyroid checkups. And I still don't feel good. This just isn't fair!" Plus your friends and family go on as if your problem does not exist, and that makes you angry. After all, it's not as if you have a "capital S" serious illness. You are not going to die from this thing. But no one seems to understand how upset you feel. You cry and feel sorry for yourself, and you find no joy in any activity. Sorrow can lead to depression and destructive feelings. Chances are, you try to bargain your way out of this problem: "If I become a vegetarian, I will be healthy again. If I lose the weight I gained from being hypothyroid, everything will go back to the way it was." Bargaining is a favorite tool of just about everybody—not only those dealing with a chronic illness. The problem with bargaining is that it does not work; it's just another name for magical thinking.

What to do The hard truth about coping with any chronic problem is that it's always there. The good news is that you will have some great days. And conversely, you will have some not so great days, depending on how you respond to treatment. Being angry about that is normal; in fact, it's healthy. It's also okay to be sad and depressed. You did not ask for this health problem, and it's okay to take some time for a little self-pity (see pages 170–171 for coping tips that can ease you through the rough days). If you find that you are dwelling on your health more than you want to, consider seeing a therapist who can help you through these stages of adjustment (see pages 126–127).

Acceptance
it doesn't happen in a day

For those with a thyroid disorder that has yet to respond to treatment, learning to accept chronic disorder as part of your life is not easy. You miss the old carefree you. You miss not having to think about your health. You now fully understand why your grandparents used to say, "Don't take your health for granted." Now you know. And with that knowledge comes a certain amount of power. It gives you back control over your life. Yes, you have this disorder, but it is treatable and it need not define who you are. You are still you, just a bit different, thanks to this chronic condition. Yes, it's a different life than the one you had originally planned before you got this problem, but that's okay. The point is to work with this new reality and make it your own. How do you do this? It's not easy. It calls for a great deal of self-exploration. Think of it as a personal journey. Social workers and therapists who have counseled people with chronic illnesses suggest the following:

Learn about your condition

For some people, becoming a student of their condition can be an important way to regain a sense of control. They feel empowered learning the new vocabulary and finding out the latest news on the Internet. But for others, reading up on their illness or surfing the Internet can be very stressful. Find your happy knowledge medium.

Get your support team together

In the beginning, it's important to find the right doctors and other support (see pages 109–130). After all, these are the people who will be helping you regain your life. You need to find doctors who will partner with you in your long-term care. Sometimes the chemistry is not right. Keep looking until you find the right doctors who can communicate effectively with you.

Try to define what you have lost and gained

Think about the pattern of your symptoms. Have they kept you from doing things you would like to do? Make a list of those things. Now think about what not doing those things means to you. Are there any alternative ways to regain, or achieve, some of what you have lost? For a lot of people with thyroid issues, fatigue and weight gain are the big hurdles. Feeling tired and being overweight can impact your exercise routine, your sex life, your work life. You need to look at how things have changed since you were diagnosed before you can make new plans. As the authors of *Recrafting Your Life* explain it, you need to "figure out which parts of [your] old life you *can* continue and which you *want* to continue."

Avoid energy-draining situations

Keeping up your energy level is vital to maintaining a sense of purpose throughout your day. Don't let anything drain it unnecessarily. Sift through your typical day. Are there any particular times or places or people that make you uncomfortable? Try to identify them and see what you can do to turn things around. For example, if you find that driving to work tires you out, consider other means of transport, such as carpooling, where you don't have to do the driving all the time. If you notice your fatigue is at its highest at the end of the day, plan on taking a rest then.

Seek spiritual renewal

Having a chronic illness can be a blessing in disguise. For one thing, it teaches you who your real friends are. They are the ones who stuck by you and continue to stick by you through thick and thin. Having a health problem can also make you cherish life more because you have learned not to take it for granted. It lets you see the bigger picture. For many, this is the first time they have ever questioned the meaning of their life. To that end, seek out books, poems, plays, and movies about people who have overcome great odds. These heroic stories can do wonders for your spirit.

Relapses

bumps along the way

You have been managing just fine, dealing with all your new physical and mental changes to the best of your ability. Good for you. And then, wham, your symptoms flare up. Maybe you have come down with another illness or some other stressor, like a bad spell at work, and it's making you feel lousy. What do you do? If you think it's stress related, you can work on cutting back on your daily stress level. If you think it's due to your thyroid condition or some other health issue, you will need to call your doctor and make an appointment. Yes, it can feel as if you are starting all over again. You are reminded of the first time you had any of these annoying symptoms. And now here you are again, still suffering. This is called having a relapse, and it is part and parcel of having a chronic illness, even if it is a nominal one like a thyroid disorder. Try to remember that having a chronic illness calls for a different way of looking at your health. You will have good days as well as bad days. And sometimes those bad days will last for a week or two or three. This lack of predictability is to be expected. If it's any comfort, you are not alone. Over half the population of America—that's 100 million people—has some kind of chronic health problem.

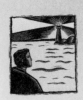

FIRST PERSON INSIGHTS

The new improved me

I was always suspicious of those stories about people who changed their lives around after they came down with some dire illness. But after my own prolonged bout with hypothyroidism, I can now appreciate those stories. Having hypothyroidism has changed my understanding of myself and my place in the world. It has taken four years to finally get my thyroid condition under control, and in those years I learned to let go of the little things. I was too tired to keep up appearances. I learned to "let go and let live." I call it my spiritual makeover.

—Sonya S., Philadelphia, PA

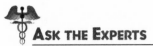

ASK THE EXPERTS

I was under a lot of stress at work, and the next thing I knew I was dealing with these terrible bouts of fatigue. My doctor upped my thyroid medicine, but I had to take a week off from work. My colleagues are now mad at me. What can I do?

It's difficult for colleagues to understand the nature of an "invisible" illness such as thyroid disease. You do not "look" ill, but inside you sometimes don't feel well. You have a choice to tell them about your condition or not. Either way, there is no need for you to apologize for taking sick days. If you need to take more than your allotted number of days, then you might want to consider talking to your supervisor about making some adjustments in your work schedule. For more on this, see pages 162–163.

I have three young children, a part-time job, and a husband who travels a lot. How do I know if my fatigue is due to my hypothyroidism or just a reflection of my daily life?

Good question. This is precisely why having a chronic health problem can be so vexing. It's hard to know the reason for your symptoms. Tracking your symptoms in your health journal (see pages 14–15) can help you see if any patterns are taking shape. If the fatigue continues for more than a week, it's a good idea to check with your doctor. It may be your thyroid. Then again, it may not.

Helpful resources

The Chronic Illness Workbook
by Pat Fennel

Recrafting a Life
by Charlie Johnson and
Denise Webster

On Death and Dying
by Elisabeth Kübler-Ross, M.D.

Illness As Metaphor
by Susan Sontag

On Being Ill
by Virginia Woolf

CHAPTER 11

Issues for Women and Children

Pregnancy and thyroid trouble
how the thyroid can make itself known

Thyroid problems are much more common in women than in men. They are also more complicated. One reason is pregnancy, a complex process that profoundly affects a woman's body, including metabolic processes of all kinds. In general, pregnancy does not cause thyroid disorders, but if they appear before, during, or after pregnancy, they can lead to medical problems for mother and child. The chances of having thyroid problems during pregnancy are extremely low. But because the disorders are potentially very harmful, doctors and their pregnant patients must take them seriously.

It's important to remember that even in a normal pregnancy, a woman can have symptoms that resemble those caused by a thyroid malfunction. The gland may swell for lack of iodine because the fetus must take its share of the element. The thyroid can also get bigger because a hormone similar to TSH (thyroid-stimulating hormone) is generated during pregnancy and stimulates the gland. A perfectly normal pregnancy can induce intolerance to heat, nervousness, fatigue, heart palpitations, and sweating—all symptoms of hyperthyroidism.

Hyperthyroidism during pregnancy is complicated by two frustrating facts: Instead of radioactive scans, doctors use physical examinations and blood tests. And because they cannot treat a pregnant woman with radioactive materials, doctors use antithyroid medication. The drugs used most often here are propylthiouracil and methimazole. The main rule for the use of such drugs is this: Use the smallest possible dose that will correct the hyperthyroidism. If a woman cannot use these drugs (if, for example, she is allergic to them), surgery to remove her thyroid gland may be the best option.

Hypothyroidism during pregnancy is easier to deal with than hyperthyroidism. Usually blood tests to detect levels of TSH can confirm the presence of the underactive thyroid, and treatment is much the same as it is in women who are not pregnant (doses of synthetic hormone).

Because of the possibly dire consequences for the mother and fetus of having thyroid trouble during pregnancy, many physicians recommend thyroid screening tests for women who are contemplating a pregnancy. Screening is especially important for women with a personal or family history of thyroid problems and women who have an autoimmune disease (for example, pernicious anemia or type 1 diabetes).

The thyroid gland and infertility

Many factors can cause infertility in women, and thyroid trouble is one of them, though it accounts for only a small percentage of cases. Here are the most important facts to remember about thyroid-related infertility:

◆ Thyroid problems affecting fertility can appear simultaneously with other conditions that also diminish fertility. In such cases, treating the thyroid trouble alone will not restore normal fertility.

◆ If a woman's infertility is caused by a thyroid disorder alone, treating the thyroid problem can correct the infertility.

◆ The extreme fatigue that thyroid problems typically cause can reduce sexual desire, making intercourse less likely.

◆ If you are having difficulty getting pregnant, ask your doctor about having your thyroid checked.

Trouble after pregnancy
keeping your thyroid on track

Your thyroid worries are not necessarily over after delivery, because thyroid disorders often occur *after* pregnancy. The three most common types are Graves' disease (an autoimmune disorder and the main cause of hyperthyroidism), Hashimoto's thyroiditis (also an autoimmune disorder and the main cause of hypothyroidism), and postpartum thyroiditis (an inflammation of the thyroid).

If you are treated for Graves' disease before getting pregnant or during pregnancy and the treatment vanquishes the disorder, you may experience the problem again after delivery. Also, your baby may become hyperthyroid, even if your thyroid condition was under control during pregnancy. There is mandatory thyroid testing for babies at birth. You, too, will need to be tested after giving birth.

Hashimoto's thyroiditis can also creep up on you after pregnancy. A postpartum blood test to check TSH and thyroxine is a prudent precaution, especially if you have an autoimmune disease or your family has a history of thyroid trouble.

Postpartum thyroiditis is the most common after-pregnancy disorder. It's an inflammation of the thyroid that can bring on mild hyperthyroidism or mild hypothyroidism. Postpartum thyroiditis is often the real cause of what some women call "the baby blues" or "postpartum depression." Postpartum depression is a common, natural outcome of delivering a baby. Postpartum thyroiditis, on the other hand, is a thyroid disorder that often results in depression and can readily be treated if it's diagnosed right after delivery. This disorder usually goes away on its own in a few weeks. When doctors treat it, they often prescribe doses of thyroid hormone or antithyroid pills.

Silent lymphocytic thyroiditis is one of the maladies included in the term *postpartum thyroiditis*. Women with postpartum silent lymphocytic thyroiditis experience both hyperthyroidism and hypothyroidism. The symptoms are typically mild and include depression, insomnia, restlessness, anxiety, poor concentration, fatigue, and weight gain.

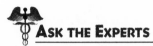

ASK THE EXPERTS

If I take antithyroid drugs to treat my postpartum Graves' disease, will they show up in my breast milk?

Not as long as the drugs are taken in minimal doses. The two most widely used antithyroid medications are propylthiouracil and methimazole. In low doses these drugs will not pass into breast milk and are therefore safe for breastfeeding.

If I have Graves' disease before pregnancy, can the condition then be passed to the fetus while I'm pregnant?

Yes. Graves' disease is an autoimmune disorder that causes thyroid-stimulating antibodies to be released into your bloodstream, leading to hyperthyroidism. These antibodies can linger around in your system even after you've been successfully treated for Graves' disease. If you later become pregnant, the leftover antibodies can pass through your placenta and trigger hyperthyroidism in the fetus. Treating the fetus, in this case, is a matter of treating the mother: Antithyroid drugs taken by the mother will pass to the fetus.

How can I tell if I'm at risk for developing postpartum thyroiditis?

Unfortunately, there are only two factors that help us gauge the risk: (1) the presence of antithyroid antibodies and (2) a family history of autoimmune thyroiditis. Having one or both of these makes you more likely to develop postpartum thyroiditis.

Thyroid concerns for women
how your thyroid disorder can affect other illnesses

Besides pregnancy, many other facets of women's health are intimately intertwined with thyroid function. Here are a few of the most important:

Heart disease is a big concern in women, just as it is in men. In fact, heart disease is the leading cause of death in women. The thyroid can be part of this mix in a couple of ways. First, because both hyperthyroidism and hypothyroidism can affect the heart (through changes in heart rate, heart rhythm, and blood pressure), they can put additional stress on a woman's cardiovascular system. Second, thyroid trouble during menopause can raise the risk of heart disease, which is naturally increased in menopause because of a drop in estrogen levels. Both hypo- and hyperthyroidism can cause cardiovascular changes that boost the risk of heart trouble throughout menopause.

Osteoporosis is a disease in which bones thin out, gradually becoming susceptible to fractures. The condition affects millions of Americans, but it hits hardest among women. The bone thinning gets worse as women age and accelerates dramatically when they enter menopause. The process of building and dismantling human bone mass goes on all the time. Old bone material is removed, and new bone material replaces it. In osteoporosis, though, bone is removed faster than it can be replaced. One thing that can speed up this bone-thinning cycle is hyperthyroidism. Fortunately, when the overactive thyroid is successfully treated, the thyroid-induced bone loss stops. However, other risk factors for osteoporosis, such as inadequate calcium intake, decreased estrogen levels, vitamin D deficiency, and lack of exercise may continue to exert their influence.

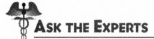

ASK THE EXPERTS

Can I safely take the Pill while I'm on synthetic thyroid hormone?

Yes. Taking thyroid hormone and an oral contraceptive is a very low-risk regimen. It's important to remember, though, that oral contraceptives themselves can have side effects that resemble those caused by thyroid dysfunctions. So it's possible to mistakenly conclude that symptoms caused by the Pill are the result of a thyroid problem or that you don't have a thyroid disorder because side effects from the oral contraceptive are disguising the thyroid problem. To avoid the confusion, you need to make sure your doctor knows that you are taking both kinds of drugs.

If I'm pregnant and have an overactive thyroid, can I wait until after delivery to be treated for the thyroid problem?

Absolutely not. Untreated hyperthyroidism can lead to hyperthyroidism in the baby, malformations in the fetus, miscarriage, stillbirth, and premature birth. Hyperthyroidism in the mother must be brought under control as soon as possible. Fortunately, overactive thyroids during pregnancy are rare.

Can thyroid problems interfere with my fertility?

Yes, both hypo- and hyperthyroidism can disrupt normal menstruation and ovulation, making conception difficult, though not impossible.

Can thyroid problems cause menstrual problems?

Menstrual problems can arise any time that thyroid hormones become unbalanced. If you are hyperthyroid, your periods may change dramatically. They may become irregular, light, or nonexistent. If you are hypothyroid, they may become heavy, long, and in severe cases completely absent. Such symptoms, of course, could also indicate conditions that have nothing to do with the thyroid. In any case, menstrual irregularities like these should be checked out by a physician.

Thyroid trouble in infants
what to look out for

Newborns can have thyroid problems just as adults can. In fact, the causes and symptoms of thyroid dysfunction in the young closely parallel those in grown-ups. But there is one big difference: The consequences of thyroid disorders in newborns are often far more serious than those in adults. Their mental functions, their physical growth, their complex development—all these processes are unfolding. And these processes are all at stake if something goes wrong. If that something is thyroid function, the impact on little bodies and brains can be far reaching because thyroid hormone touches virtually every cell.

Without the right amount of thyroid hormone, the fetus can become hypo- or hyperthyroid. The harm done can include poor bone development, above-normal heart rate, low birth weight, impaired hearing, heart failure, small head size, below-normal mental function, and breathing trouble. Newborns and children with thyroid disorders may have a goiter, low birth weight, stunted growth, low body temperature, bulging or prominent eyes, mental retardation, rapid heartbeat, and misshapen heads. As they get older, they may be unusually fretful, tired, sweaty, or emotional. Children and teens may have many symptoms, including poor growth, excessive fatigue, poor concentration, underdeveloped bones and teeth, slow pulse, brittle nails, and heat intolerance.

The silver lining here is that screening tests can easily detect thyroid problems in newborns. Since the 1970s, screening tests for newborns have been required by law in the United States. When babies are treated, they usually respond quickly, avoiding the dangerous consequences that arise down the line. With treatment, many signs and symptoms can be reversed.

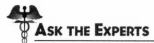

Ask the Experts

How can I tell if my newborn has hypothyroidism?

Hypothyroid newborns often have no obvious signs or symptoms of hypothyroidism, so testing is the only way to be sure about the diagnosis. If the baby has an extreme case of underactive thyroid, however, some signs can be more pronounced: slow pulse, difficulty feeding, and protrusion of the belly button, also known as umbilical hernia.

My baby was diagnosed with hypothyroidism at birth. Does this mean that she will have brain damage?

Many babies are born with hypothyroidism. But if these babies are given synthetic thyroid hormone therapy, they will be free of any permanent damage.

Normal Thyroid Development in Children	
10 weeks of gestation	thyroid gland begins to work
12 weeks	TSH present
12 weeks	thyroid hormones present
18–36 weeks	thyroid hormones increase
at birth	temporary surge in thyroid hormones
after birth	thyroid hormones affect organs

Hyperthyroidism in children
more energy than necessary

Hyperthyroidism can occur weeks before a baby is born. The condition, though, is usually temporary and rare. Overactive thyroids are also rare in children up to age five. Prenatal hyperthyroidism is triggered by thyroid-stimulating antibodies that pass through the placenta from the mother. That is, it happens because the mother has Graves' disease. Fortunately, hyperthyroidism shows up only in babies whose mothers have extremely potent antibodies. Such antibodies are present in just 1 to 2 percent of mothers with Graves' disease, resulting in hyperthyroidism in about 1 in 50,000 newborns.

The biochemical dance between mother and fetus is complicated. If the mother is treated with antithyroid drugs during pregnancy, the baby is unlikely to be hyperthyroid. Antithyroid drugs pass through the placenta and treat the fetus as well as the mother. But if the mother does not have hyperthyroidism but does harbor thyroid-stimulating antibodies left over from a previous bout of hyperthyroidism, the baby can end up being hyperthyroid. Sometimes, because of the complex biochemistry going on in the infant, hyperthyroidism doesn't appear for one or two months after birth. In fact, such intricacies can lead to an even more unusual situation: hyperthyroidism occurring in babies born to hypothyroid mothers.

Doctors suspect hyperthyroidism in the fetus when the heart rate is 160 beats per minute. In newborns, the signs and symptoms include fast heartbeat, irritability, inadequate weight gain, goiter, and bulging eyes. If hyperthyroidism is not properly treated, it can cause irregular heartbeat, heart failure, and, in extreme cases, death. Untreated hyperthyroidism in both the fetus and the newborn can also have long-term effects: misshapen skull, inadequate growth, and delayed development.

Doctors treat hyperthyroid fetuses by giving the mother antithyroid drugs. They also treat newborns and children under five with antithyroid medication, which almost always does its job in three to six weeks. Sometimes physicians use nonradioactive iodine if the hyperthyroidism is severe. With infants, surgery and radioactive iodine are almost never appropriate.

Children can get Graves' disease, though usually not until the age of 12. They generally have the same symptoms that adults do: prominent or bulging eyes, heart palpitations, nervousness, irritability, exhaustion, restlessness, excessive sweating, insomnia, and heat intolerance. Many of these symptoms can be barely noticeable, but an alert parent can usually pick up on them. Some parents, however, may miss the clues and blame the symptoms on behavior problems or attention deficit disorder (ADD). Before treating for ADD, it's a good idea to have your child checked for thyroid disorders, especially if they run in your family. Diagnosis requires just a physical examination and a thyroid-function blood test.

FIRST PERSON INSIGHTS

It wasn't ADD

The trouble started when my son began third grade. He was always an energetic boy, but now he couldn't contain it and was fidgety and cranky in class. At home he complained of being tired. I chalked it up to normal school-adjustment problems. But then his concentration was off and he would get very upset over the least little thing. He wasn't sleeping well, and he even started wetting the bed again. I was frantic. The school psychologist thought he might have ADD. I thought he should have a complete physical before we did anything. Turns out he had Graves' disease. His doctor thought it might have developed after he had a bad bout of strep throat a year ago. The good news is that the medication has taken care of all his symptoms and he is back to being himself again. What an ordeal. Thank goodness his doctor checked him from head to toe.

—Simone F., Narrowsburg, NY

Hypothyroidism in children
too slow and tired

When babies are born with an underactive thyroid, they are said to have congenital hypothyroidism. In North America, about 1 in every 4,000 babies are born with the disorder. Most cases of congenital hypothyroidism (about 80 to 85 percent) are caused by structural flaws in the thyroid—a thyroid that is shrunken, located in the wrong place in the neck, or missing altogether. Iodine deficiency in the mother, which is common in many parts of the world, is the main reason for this thyroid problem. Other causes include metabolic problems, such as the thyroid's failure to produce hormone or to react to TSH. Also, if the mother is exposed to radioactive iodine during pregnancy, the baby's thyroid can be damaged or destroyed.

A baby with congenital hypothyroidism may have several signs and symptoms, such as jaundice, constipation, inadequate feeding, decreased crying, umbilical hernia, and cool skin. But these signs can be subtle and easily missed. The damage that hypothyroidism can do, though, is not so low key. If left untreated, congenital hypothyroidism can cause mental retardation and stunted physical growth. Ignoring a baby's hypothyroidism for a month or more can be disastrous. Mental or physical impairment is sure to occur.

Fortunately, mandatory screening tests can detect hypothyroidism in newborns. This screening, a simple blood test done a couple of days after birth, usually catches hypothyroidism before any permanent damage can be done.

If the baby is found to have hypothyroidism, treatment begins right away. Initial treatment consists of daily doses of synthetic thyroid hormone. Later the dosage may change depending on the outcome of regular testing of the baby's thyroid function. If proper treatment is given early enough, it can block mental retardation and growth problems.

Hypothyroidism in children is not always congenital. Sometimes it's acquired and can show up years later to impede growth and development. In countries where iodine is readily available, the main cause of underactive thyroid in children is autoimmune thyroiditis, an inflammation of the thyroid gland. This disorder appears more often in girls than in boys and more frequently in those with a family history of autoimmune thyroid disease.

The treatment for childhood hypothyroidism is synthetic thyroid hormone, carefully calibrated to the child's metabolic needs. This adjusting of hormone doses is important, because giving too much hormone can be harmful, just as giving too little is. But if the right dose is given, growth impairment can actually be reversed.

Symptoms of childhood hypothyroidism

Congenital hypothyroidism	Acquired hypothyroidism
jaundice	goiter
constipation	stunted physical growth
inadequate feeding	fatigue, lack of energy
decreased crying	cool and dry skin
umbilical hernia	brittle nails
cool, dry skin	slow pulse
mental retardation	hoarseness
stunted physical growth	slow speech
slow pulse	obesity
	cold intolerance
	swelling

Goiters in children
dealing with little lumps

The most obvious sign that a child has a thyroid disorder is a protruding goiter, a noticeable bulge in the neck. In North America, goiter is also the most common thyroid condition in school-age children, especially girls. The chief cause of an enlarged thyroid gland is autoimmune thyroiditis, which can lead to hypothyroidism. Usually when these goiters appear they show up alone, without other symptoms. In fact, most children with goiter have normally functioning thyroids. Even without symptoms, however, the enlarged area on the neck is often enough of a clue to alert doctors and parents to the condition. Any lumps need to be checked out by a doctor. Usually, they are nearly all benign, as thyroid cancer in children is very rare.

Multinodular goiters, or enlarged thyroids with nodules, are the second most common kind of goiter. They are not caused by autoimmune thyroiditis. In fact, their exact cause is unknown, though some experts think that there must be an autoimmune process that results in this kind of thyroid enlargement. Multinodular goiters also behave differently from thyroiditis-type goiters. Many of them get smaller without treatment. Others may expand and shrink repeatedly. Doctors try to distinguish between multinodular goiters and the thyroiditis-type goiters because there is a high risk of developing hypothyroidism with the thyroiditis type, but not the multinodular variety.

Doses of thyroid hormone are unlikely to shrink them. Part of the reason is that such goiters are produced by thyroids that are already functioning correctly. If the enlarged thyroids are pressing against the esophagus and other structures in the neck or if the goiters are disfiguring, many doctors will surgically remove the goiters or treat them with radioactive iodine.

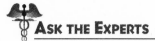# ASK THE EXPERTS

Are goiters in children painful?

In most cases, no. The most common type of goiter in children is caused by autoimmune thyroiditis. This kind is asymptomatic, meaning there are no other symptoms, including pain. Children with an asymptomatic goiter may have difficulty swallowing if the goiter grows large enough to press against structures in the neck, but pain is unlikely. A rare type of goiter caused by acute or subacute thyroiditis, however, can be painful.

Are goiters in children rare?

Actually, they occur more often than most people realize. The incidence of goiter in school-age children is 4 to 6 percent. Among these kids with goiter, girls outnumber boys by as much as a 3 to 1 margin. Affected girls are likely to get goiters around puberty.

If there are no symptoms, how can doctors tell the difference between the most common type of goiter and a multinodular goiter?

The distinction usually cannot be made just by feeling the goiter. Thyroid function blood tests, though, can tell the tale. Thyroid-antibody tests can reveal whether the goiter is caused by autoimmune thyroiditis. A positive test result suggests the common type of goiter. Tests to check for levels of TSH and thyroid hormone can show whether thyroid function is normal. Normal thyroid function also points to common goiter.

Isn't it dangerous to use radioactive iodine to treat children who have cancer?

No. Research suggests that radioactive iodine is a fairly benign treatment. As with other standard treatments for cancer in children, the benefits of radioactive iodine greatly outweigh the possible risks.

Helpful resources

*Thyroid Problems in Women and
Children*
by Joan Gomez, M.D.

**Thyroid Foundation of
America, Inc.**
Tel: 800 832-8321
Fax: 617 534-1515
www.allthyroid.org

**American Foundation of Thyroid
Patients**
Tel: 432 694-9966
www.thyroidfoundation.org

*Merck Manual of Medical
Information*
www.merck.com

Gland Central
(Internet source of thyroid
information)
www.glandcentral.com

CHAPTER 12

Thyroid Problems after 60

The older thyroid
the effect of aging on the thyroid

When it comes to thyroid disorders in older people, the biggest source of confusion is that many of the thyroid symptoms also arise during the normal process of aging. Hyperthyroidism and normal aging can both cause fatigue, weight loss, muscle wasting, excessive sweating, irregular heartbeat, tremor, heart failure, and weakness. Hypothyroid seniors may experience hoarseness, deafness, muscle cramps, anemia, constipation, low body temperature, dry skin, cold intolerance, weakness in the hands, and weight gain—all classic signs and symptoms of getting older. Such hypothyroid symptoms are general enough and vague enough to be associated with many other diseases, including depression, Parkinson's disease, type 1 diabetes, and pernicious anemia. Now add to this confusion the fact that thyroid trouble is fairly common in seniors.

Here's what you need to know about thyroid problems after age 60:

1. Symptoms may be entirely different from those in younger people.
2. Symptoms may be overlooked or thought to be normal by the very people who are experiencing them.
3. Progression of thyroid disorders in older bodies may be very different from the course of the illness in younger bodies.
4. Thyroid problems are often confused with other diseases.
5. Thyroid dysfunction in older people is much harder to detect than it is at younger ages.

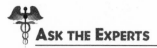
I heard that the thyroid blood test is not that good at detecting thyroid problems in seniors. Why is that?

The typical TSH blood screening test will readily tell if you are having a thyroid problem, regardless of your age. The problem lies with drug interactions that can give a false reading. A number of drugs that seniors commonly take, such as heparin (a blood thinner) and corticosteroids (for joint problems) can give false TSH readings. Always tell your doctor what medications you are on before you have a thyroid blood test.

I'm turning 60 next year. How often should I have my thyroid tested?

Because thyroid disorders are fairly common among the senior population, doctors advise testing for thyroid problems every year.

FIRST PERSON INSIGHTS

Everything changes with age

My mother had Graves' disease as a young woman. It was awful. I remember how nervous she was and how she ate all the time even though she was skin and bones. When they finally diagnosed her it was almost too late. When I turned 65 and got on Medicaid, I went for a checkup with the new doctor at the clinic. When I mentioned that my mother had had Graves' disease, this doctor ordered a thyroid check. I told him that wasn't necessary because I didn't have any symptoms. In fact, I had no appetite and was sleeping like a baby. I had even started to take naps in the afternoon. I figured it was just another sign of aging. The blood tests came back and boy, was I surprised to learn that I had hypothyroidism. My doctor told me that after a certain age, thyroid symptoms can change.

—Michael K., Duck, NC

Hyperthyroidism at 60 plus
why treatment is a bit different

Treating older people with thyroid disease is similar to treating younger people with the illness. The main differences are that physicians must take into account any other diseases that seniors might have as well as the fact that seniors are typically more sensitive to thyroid treatments than young people are.

The primary treatment for hyperthyroidism in this age group is radioactive iodine. The iodine damages the thyroid so that it stops overproducing thyroid hormone. Sometimes, though, physicians use antithyroid drugs for a few weeks before administering the iodine. The purpose is to slow down an overactive thyroid that might suddenly spill thyroid hormone into the bloodstream when the thyroid is damaged by the iodine.

For seniors, radioactive iodine is safe, effective, and fast. One dose of iodine, taken orally, can force hormone levels back to normal, reining in the overacting thyroid. The process can take as little as four weeks. After your hormone levels fall in line, you'll need to have them checked every few months. The main side effect of this treatment is hypothyroidism. Within the first year of treatment, the damaged thyroid will stop producing adequate amounts of thyroid hormone. This artificially induced hypothyroidism occurs in both young and old and is an almost unavoidable result of curing the hyperthyroidism. The hypothyroidism must then be treated for life with daily doses of synthetic hormone. And, of course, continuous treatment requires long-term monitoring of thyroid-hormone levels.

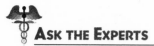

Ask the Experts

Can surgery be used to treat hyperthyroidism in seniors?

Surgery is rarely used for this purpose. Most of the time, antithyroid drugs plus radioactive iodine are the treatments of choice for an overactive thyroid. If, however, an enlarged thyroid gland is pressing against the windpipe and other structures in the neck, or nodules need to be removed, surgery is the best bet.

Do antithyroid drugs have side effects?

Just like any other drug, antithyroid medications can produce side effects. They can cause hives, rashes, joint pain, fever, and lowering of the white blood cell count. Because of these possible problems, many doctors prefer to treat seniors with radioactive iodine alone.

What other drugs do doctors use for an overactive thyroid?

To lessen the discomfort of symptoms, sometimes physicians prescribe beta-blocker medications, such as propranolol. As their name suggests, these drugs block the effect of thyroid hormone on various tissues. They may also help to prepare the way for radioactive iodine therapy by controlling symptoms.

Hypothyroidism at 60 plus

taking action early

Hypothyroidism in older people can take on two different forms. Fully developed hypothyroidism can arise, bringing with it the typical hypothyroid symptoms. But a very mild form called **subclinical hypothyroidism** can also occur without causing any obvious symptoms. The only sign of this condition is an increased blood level of TSH. Normally, people with full-blown hypothyroidism have elevated blood levels of TSH and low levels of thyroid hormone. But in subclinical hypothyroidism, TSH is high and thyroid hormone is normal, signs that the thyroid gland is starting to fail. The probability that a case of subclinical hypothyroidism will turn into full hypothyroidism is highest if the patient has both high TSH and antithyroid antibodies.

Physicians respond to subclinical hypothyroidism in different ways. Some monitor the condition and administer synthetic thyroid hormone only if hypothyroid symptoms appear. Others treat people with the condition even though no symptoms are present, because research suggests that some of these patients feel better after taking thyroid hormone. And some doctors treat people with subclinical hypothyroidism because they believe that doing so will lower the patient's risk of Alzheimer's disease.

Treatment for obvious hypothyroidism is more straightforward—it simply consists of daily doses of synthetic hormone. But as with any kind of hypothyroidism in seniors, hormone treatment should start out at very low doses and progress slowly to higher ones. Older people require less synthetic hormone than younger folks, in part because synthetic hormone stays longer in older systems. Too much hormone can also cause heart-related symptoms, such as angina, fast pulse, and irregular heartbeat.

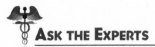

I have atrial fibrillation and my doctor wants to check me out for thyroid problems. Why is that?

Atrial fibrillation, or irregular heartbeat, can be a sign of hyperthyroidism. Moreover, amiodarone, the drug used to treat it, can cause both hyper- and hypothyroidism.

What can I do to ensure that my doctor does not miss any thyroid disease?

First, talk to your doctor about your concerns and be sure to mention any relevant information (for example, details on any symptoms you might have and whether thyroid trouble runs in your family). Second, request a thyroid function test.

Signs of hypothyroidism in seniors that are easily overlooked

grooved nails	weight gain	cold intolerance
dry skin	constipation	thinning out of skin
congestive heart failure	loss of hair	changes in mental functioning
lung infections	lethargy	

Thyroid nodules in seniors
they can happen at any age

Probably the most important lessons to learn about thyroid nodules in older people are:

1. Nodules are common in seniors.

2. Thyroid cancer is rare in seniors.

In other words, nodules in older people are not as worrisome as they are in younger people, so treatment in seniors is not as aggressive as it often is in those under age 60. To doctors, this low-risk situation means that they should try very hard to avoid doing surgery to determine if a nodule is malignant. They think, why subject a patient to surgery when it's probably not necessary?

Instead of doing surgery, doctors take a less radical path. Thyroid nodules in seniors are often not treated at all if levels of thyroid hormone are normal and if the nodules appear to be functioning normally. A radioactive iodine scan can reveal whether the nodules are functioning as usual. The scan tells the tale, because benign thyroid nodules can absorb radioactive iodine, just as the gland itself can, but malignant nodules cannot absorb it. Sometimes the iodine scan is combined with an ultrasound test. An ultrasound picture can show whether the nodules are cysts (that is, lumps filled with fluid). Thyroid cysts are benign.

If these tests suggest that a nodule is not functioning, doctors will probably want to do a fine-needle biopsy to get a sample of tissue to check microscopically for abnormal cells. In most cases involving seniors, the biopsy shows that the nodules are benign. In instances in which the nodules are shown to be cancerous or extremely suspicious, surgery is the best way to get rid of them. Believe it or not, even in older patients thyroid surgery is low risk, and postoperative recovery is fast.

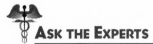

ASK THE EXPERTS

What causes hyperthyroidism after age 60?

The main causes are Graves' disease (the primary cause of hyperthyroidism), thyroiditis (an inflammation of the thyroid gland), multinodular goiter (thyroid gland with several nodules), and solitary toxic adenoma (a benign growth that mimics thyroid function).

Are there diseases or conditions that can skew thyroid function tests?

Yes. Many serious illnesses can decrease levels of thyroid hormone, producing a reading that seems to indicate hypothyroidism. Some conditions are common in older people, and these are often the ones that can scramble thyroid tests. For example, both diabetes and liver disease exert an influence, and so can malnutrition, a prevalent condition among many seniors.

I'm 61 years old and taking synthetic thyroid hormone. My hypothyroidism has been under control for months. So why do I have to keep going back to the doctor for yet another thyroid test?

Many factors can change your thyroid's requirement for thyroid hormone over time. The very process of aging can alter your hormone needs and prompt a change in your hormone dosage. Just getting your dosage of hormone properly calibrated can require several thyroid tests over the span of a year or more. The growth of a new nodule, radioactive iodine therapy, and nonthyroid medications can all prompt a change in how your body absorbs the synthetic hormone.

Helpful resources

**ThyCa: Thyroid Cancer Survivors'
Association, Inc.**
www.thyca.org

Gland Central
www.glandcentral.com

Thyroid Foundation of Canada
www.thyroid.ca

**Thyroid-Cancer.net
The Johns Hopkins Thyroid
Tumor Center**
www.thyroid-cancer.net

American Thyroid Association
www.thyroid.org

Cutting-Edge Research

Advances in testing
new blood tests

In recent years, scientists have started using an expanded range of super-sensitive blood tests that can detect even the slightest bit of thyroid imbalance. This is a great boon to people who have suffered from thyroid dysfunction for years but have always had "normal" results based on the traditional thyroid panel of blood tests. The old thyroid panel includes tests that measure T_4 and T_3 (total triiodothyronine), TSH (thyroid-stimulating hormone), FT_4 (free T_4), and T_3 and T_4 resin uptake. All of these tests measure different aspects of thyroid function, but critics say they do not give a complete picture, especially when it comes to T_3, the hormone that gives our bodies energy. It is this thyroid hormone that scientists believe plays a major role in regulating mood and mental functioning.

The new thyroid panel goes further. Among other things, it tests for free or unbound T_3, or the amount of T_3 that is actually floating around in the bloodstream. This test allows doctors to better treat patients who had "normal" test results using the old thyroid test panel but still reported symptoms of hypothyroidism—that is, fatigue, brain fog, memory problems, and low libido.

The bottom line: If you are one of the many people with normal TSH or thyroid-panel results but still feel that you have symptoms of a thyroid disorder, it may be worth it to do some research on the new blood tests and then try to find a doctor who will administer them.

Do you need T₃ therapy?

Synthroid is synthetic T_4 hormone. When you take it, your body will convert some of that T_4 into T_3. Some researchers question the efficacy of this conversion process. If you are like many hypothyroid people who are taking a synthetic T_4 replacement alone and still don't feel 100 percent, take this quiz on the possible mental side effects of low T_3. If most of these statements apply to you, it could be that you are suffering from low T_3 levels. Many people who have gone on T_3 therapy report that it has turned their lives around, and they only wish they had known about it sooner. So, do not delay in having your T_3 levels checked out if you think you might benefit.

If you have been tested for thyroid problems and you suffer from the majority of these symptoms, you could be suffering from undiagnosed hypothyroidism. Take a look at the full symptom checklist for hypothyroidism in Chapter 1. Then see your doctor and get tested.

Beware that both subclinical hypothyroidism and hypothyroidism are often misdiagnosed as depression, so do push to have the full set of tests done and then discuss the results with your doctor. See your doctor if you answer "yes" to any of these questions:

- I am unable to concentrate for long periods of time.
- I feel confused and like my mind is in a fog.
- I feel depressed for no reason.
- I am moodier than usual.
- I am more forgetful than usual.
- I have feelings of worthlessness.
- I feel extremely lethargic, sometimes unable to get out of my chair.
- I have lost interest in everyday activities.
- I feel like there is no reason to wake up in the morning.
- My sex drive has decreased or I am having other sexual problems.

The new guidelines for TSH
lower ranges are now used

Prior to 2001, anyone with a TSH level between .05 and 5 mlU/L (micro units per milliliter of blood), or even up to 10 mlU/L, was thought to have a healthy thyroid, even if he or she complained of the usual symptoms of thyroid disorder. But in 2001 the American Association of Clinical Endocrinologists (AACE) suggested that the normal TSH range should be narrowed to just .03 to 3 mlU/L. The AACE stated that people with a TSH level in the gray area between .03 and .05 mlU/L most likely suffer from a thyroid disorder.

The impact of these lower guidelines on thyroid medicine is enormous. For one thing, these new guidelines now put the number of Americans with some form of hypothyroidism at 27 million (instead of 10 million). This makes thyroid disorders one of the major health problems in America.

What this really signifies is that more people need to be tested for possible thyroid disorders. Before this guideline change, the basic thyroid panel was usually administered only to people with major risk factors or people who complained of symptoms of thyroid disorder. Now the American Thyroid Association suggests that people have their TSH levels tested every five years after age 35. At the other extreme, some doctors are beginning to think TSH tests are misleading and should be scrapped. They believe the real deciding factor in thyroid illness is the presence of antithyroid antibodies, which are used to indicate the two autoimmune thyroid diseases, Graves' (see page 34) and Hashimoto's (see page 38).

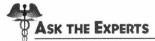

My TSH level is 4, which is apparently a sign of mild thyroid failure, but I have no symptoms. Should I be taking medication?

Your doctor will need to make that call, based on your risk of developing full-blown hypothyroidism later on. If you fall into any of the risk categories below, your doctor may consider starting you on a low-dose trial of hormone-replacement therapy:

- Female, Caucasian, and/or elderly
- Family history of thyroid disease
- High cholesterol level
- Diabetes diagnosis
- Pregnancy or postpartum status
- Treatment for thyroid problems in the past
- Presence of another autoimmune disease
- On medication for bipolar disorder
- Smoker

FIRST PERSON INSIGHTS

How I became an advocate

After I was diagnosed with Graves', I headed for the library computer and read everything I could find on it. I came across the American Foundation of Thyroid Patients. It has online articles that focus on taking care of your thyroid and information on new research. The more I read, the more interested I became. When I got home, I picked up the phone and called one of the nonprofit thyroid research organizations. They put me in touch with their volunteer office. By then I had done so much reading, they asked me to help in our local city chapter. I was delighted! It's been wonderful being able to share information with others.

—Joe R., Scottsdale, AZ

Thyroid-cancer advances
new findings in the war against cancer

Although the success rate in curing thyroid cancer is one of the highest in the cancer field, it is still the subject of much research because of the vital role the thyroid plays in relation to all the other organs and systems of the body. One of the most important advances is the PET scan, which enables doctors to pinpoint more accurately any cancer cells remaining after treatment. Before PET was developed, doctors could use an RAI scan to detect leftover active thyroid tissue, but they could not determine whether it was making thyroid hormone or cancer cells. They had to resort to biopsies. The PET scan can distinguish between the two without any invasive procedures.

Another important breakthrough in this area is using recombinant TSH (TSH that has been recombined with DNA material) to stimulate iodine intake. Iodine uptake is necessary for doing an RAI scan to check for remaining cancer. In order to get good test results, patients who were on thyroid-hormone therapy had to stop taking it for several weeks until they became hypothyroid. This would allow the iodine uptake test to measure their thyroid more accurately. Doctors were always concerned that, during these weeks off medication, if there was any remaining cancer it might grow more quickly. But by giving patients recombinant TSH they can do an RAI scan much sooner, and patients do not have to stop taking their hormones.

In terms of treatment, one recent advance is linked to the fact that doctors have finally figured out why women get thyroid cancer more often than men. It turns out that estrogen, which women produce in greater quantities than men, promotes the growth of some thyroid-cancer tumors. Doctors have found that giving patients an estrogen-blocking medication can slow down this growth.

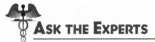

I have a thyroid tumor, but the RAI test was inconclusive for cancer, so the doctor wants to remove it. Aren't there any new ways to diagnose thyroid cancer besides surgery?

Yes. But first, your situation is common: Most doctors use RAI and fine-needle aspiration (FNA) to investigate suspicious tumors, but because these tests are often inconclusive, they usually resort to surgery to remove the tumor for testing. Most of the time, the surgery turns out to have been unnecessary because the tumor is benign. But help may be on the way. In a 2000 issue of *Science*, researchers reported on the discovery of "fusion genes" in follicular-cancer tumors and nodules (one of the four kinds of thyroid cancer). Now doctors should only have to use FNA to check for the presence of these fusion genes, avoiding invasive and unnecessary surgery.

Thyroid cancer runs in my family. Are doctors making any headway in predicting whether or not people like me will get it?

Yes indeed. When it comes to predicting thyroid cancer, researchers in Iceland discovered in 2000 that thyroglobulin can be found in the blood of people up to 15 years before they develop thyroid cancer. This is even more reason to have a thyroid-binding globulin (TBG) test done when you have your thyroid tested. And since you fall into the high-risk category for hereditary thyroid cancer, those tests should probably be done every couple of years after age 30.

Findings about other illnesses
how thyroid disorders affect other diseases

For decades, researchers have known that thyroid disorders can lead to a host of other illnesses, some life threatening. In recent years, researchers have learned even more about the effects of thyroid imbalance on the body, and these findings are likely to be even more helpful when it comes to predicting the evolution of your thyroid condition.

Heart Disease

Some of the most serious—and most common—conditions linked to hypothyroidism, in particular, are heart and circulatory problems. And not just atherosclerosis but other conditions, including uneven heart rhythm and heart rate, high blood pressure, high cholesterol, and chest pain. Atrial fibrillation can cause hyperthyroidism. Thyroid conditions can also impair the flexibility of the small arteries and reduce the force of heart-muscle contractions. New findings show that even people with subclinical hypothyroidism are at risk for heart problems, especially female patients over 50, who are three times more likely to have heart attacks than women with no thyroid problems.

Osteoporosis

There have also been some discoveries concerning osteoporosis. It was already known that postmenopausal women on T$_4$ therapy can expect accelerated bone loss, which leads to osteoporosis. Doctors have recently learned that people with hypothyroidism are also at risk for this. The same is true for hyperthyroid people who have had thyroid surgery, because this surgery often damages the parathyroid glands, which regulate calcium and, therefore, bone density.

Fibromyalgia and Chronic Fatigue Syndrome

For some 12 percent of all people diagnosed with fibromyalgia, the cause is hypothyroidism. There is also a strong correlation between chronic fatigue syndrome (CFS) and hypothyroidism. This makes sense when you realize that these three disorders share a great many symptoms: fatigue, poor sleep, brain fog, muscle weakness, and depression. There are no fast and sure diagnostic tests for these two disorders, but a simple TSH blood test will rule out hypothyroidism. The question as to whether the hypothyroidism triggers fibromyalgia or CFS or vice versa remains to be answered.

Getting into a clinical trial

put yourself in the thick of the latest thyroid research

If you are someone who has a great interest in learning more about cutting-edge thyroid research, one way to do this is to participate in a clinical trial at a major research institute or hospital. These trials are usually sponsored by the government or medical foundations and are run by researchers to test new methods of treating chronic thyroid disorders. These trials may require that you stay in a hospital (an inpatient trial) or simply visit a clinic every few weeks (outpatient trial).

There are four kinds of clinical trials:

Treatment trials examine new ways of treating illness, new combinations of drugs, or new kinds of surgery.

Prevention trials investigate ways to prevent illnesses from occurring. Such trials can involve vaccines, vitamins, medicines, or lifestyle changes.

Screening trials look for better ways to diagnose illnesses.

Quality-of-life trials are aimed at finding ways to improve comfort for people living with chronic diseases.

What are the benefits of joining a clinical trial? They include being able to take an active role in managing your health, having access to new medical treatments before everyone else, getting medical care from leading experts and top medical facilities, and making a contribution to medical research to help others like you. The risks? Since the techniques and treatments are new, there may be some unexpected and possibly serious side effects, or they may not work at all. Getting involved in a study may also mean making more of a time commitment than seeking standard treatment. Your doctor can refer you to clinical trials.

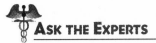

ASK THE EXPERTS

A research hospital near me is doing an interesting clinical trial on thyroid-cancer vaccines. What should I ask to determine if I can participate?

You should prepare for this visit as you would for a visit to any doctor (see page 117). Prepare a list of questions ahead of time, such as:

- ◆ What is the purpose of the study, and who will be in it?
- ◆ What kinds of tests and treatments are involved?
- ◆ Has this treatment been tested before?
- ◆ What are the possible risks, side effects, and benefits?
- ◆ How long will the trial last, and will I need to be hospitalized?
- ◆ Will I be reimbursed for any expenses or time off work?
- ◆ Will I be able to find out the results of the trial?
- ◆ Will any follow-up care be available?

And before you sign any consent forms, make sure to read the protocol (the plan for the study) from cover to cover. And remember that even after you sign the form, you can withdraw from the trial at any time.

Are clinical trials for thyroid disorders different from others?

Not necessarily. Clinical trials for thyroid disorders, like other trials, usually focus on new medications, treatments for thyroid cancer, and new diagnostic and testing techniques. And like other trials, they usually include four different phases. Find out which phase you would be in.

Phase 1 New drugs or treatments tested for the first time on a small group of people (20 to 80) to evaluate safety and identify side effects.

Phase 2 Further testing, this time on a larger group of people (100+), to see if the treatment is effective.

Phase 3 Testing on an even larger group (1,000 or more) to confirm effectiveness and compare it to other treatments.

Phase 4 Postmarketing studies to collect information on the risks, benefits, and dosage (if it's a medication).

Helpful resources

The Thyroid Sourcebook
by M. Sara Rosenthal

*The Thyroid Solution: A
Revolutionary Mind-Body Program
That Will Help You*
by Ridha Arem, M.D.

Living Well with Hypothyroidism
by Mary J. Shomon

Thyroid Balance
by Glenn S. Rothfeld, M.D., M.Ac.,
and Deborah S. Romaine

*Thyroid Power: 10 Steps to Total
Health*
by Richard L. Shames, M.D., and
Karilee Halo Shames, R.N., Ph.D.

www.clinicaltrials.gov
All you need to know about joining
a trial. You can search for thyroid
trials.

www.cc.nih.gov
Clinical trials run by the National
Institutes of Health

**American Foundation of
Thyroid Patients
Tel: 432 694-9966
www.thyroidfoundation.org**

Glossary

Words in bold type are defined elsewhere in the glossary.

antithyroid drugs Medications such as carbimazole, methimazole, and propylthiouracil that treat hyperthyroidism by reducing or preventing the production of thyroid hormone or by making it difficult for the gland to absorb iodine. See also: Thyroid-hormone replacement.

autoimmune disease An illness in which the body's defense systems perceive normal cells or tissues as disease-producing (pathogenic) cells and attack them.

beta-blockers A colloquial name for beta-adrenergic blocking agents such as propranolol. These drugs inhibit the activity of the sympathetic nervous system and certain hormones and help to relieve the symptoms of hyperthyroidism.

biopsy A small piece of tissue extracted for diagnostic purposes. A thyroid biopsy may be made by fine-needle aspiration or during surgery.

calcitonin A hormone secreted by cells that reside in the thyroid gland but that are not of thyroid origin. Measuring the calcitonin level of a person with **medullary-cell cancer** helps evaluate the effectiveness of treatment.

cold nodule A nodule in the thyroid gland that does not absorb radioisotopes during diagnostic tests or treatment. See also: Hot nodule.

cyst A closed sac or pouch with a distinct membrane that is filled with fluid, semifluid, or solid material. Cysts are usually abnormal—that is, they arise from an infection, an obstructed duct, or a developmental anomaly—and benign.

de Quervain's thyroiditis Inflammation of the thyroid gland due to a virus. Also called subacute viral thyroiditis or viral thyroiditis.

diffuse toxic goiter See: Graves' disease.

endocrinologist A medical specialist whose focus is the endocrine glands (thyroid, parathyroid, pituitary, hypothalamus, pancreas, adrenals, and the gonads) and the biochemistry of hormones.

euthyroid Having a normally functioning thyroid gland. (The prefix *eu-* means "well," "easily," or "good.") Euthyroid is also the proprietary name of a drug used to treat hypothyroidism.

free T$_3$ test A thyroid function test that measures the amount of biologically active triiodothyronine (T$_3$) in the blood. This is the T$_3$ that is not bound to a carrier protein such as thyroid-binding globulin. A free T$_3$ test is particularly helpful in diagnosing hyperthyroidism, because T$_3$ levels may rise weeks or months before the T$_4$ levels do. Low free T$_3$ levels may occur in other, nonthyroidal illnesses. See also: Free T$_4$ test.

free T$_4$ levels determine your thyroid status. The more severe the hyperthyroidism, the higher will be the free T$_4$ level; the more severe the hypothyroidism, the lower the free T$_4$. Low free T$_4$ levels may also occur in other, nonthyroidal illnesses, and misleading results sometimes arise due to the presence of certain antibodies or an unusual carrier protein in the blood. See also: Free T$_3$ test.

free T$_4$ test A thyroid function test that measures the amount of biologically active thyroxine (T$_4$) in the blood. This is the T$_4$ that is not bound to a carrier protein such as thyroid-binding globulin.

free thyroxine index This is not really a test but rather a calculation based on information from the total T$_4$ and T$_3$-resin-binding tests. Prior to the development of the free T$_4$ and free T$_3$ assays, it was used to estimate the amount of biologically active T$_4$ in the blood.

goiter Any enlargement of the thyroid gland. The gland may be so enlarged that the front of the neck appears swollen.

Graves' disease A common form of hyperthyroidism caused by overactivity of the **entire thyroid gland.** It is an autoimmune disease characterized by goiter and, often, a slight protrusion of the eyeballs. Graves' disease is sometimes called "diffuse toxic goiter."

Graves' ophthalmopathy See: Oculomotor muscles.

Hashimoto's thyroiditis An autoimmune disease that begins with inflammation and goiter and progresses to destruction of the thyroid gland and hypothyroidism. It affects women more than men and requires **thyroid-hormone replacement.**

Hashitoxicosis An episode of **hyperthyroidism** in a patient with **Hashimoto's thyroiditis**.

hormone A biochemical substance that is made in an organ, gland, or body part and secreted into the blood to produce specific effects elsewhere in the body. Hormones stimulate the increase or decrease of functional activity (such as growth or digestion) or the secretion of other hormones.

hot nodule A nodule in the **thyroid gland** that absorbs radioisotopes to a greater degree than does the surrounding normal thyroid tissue during diagnostic tests or treatment. See also: Cold nodule.

Hyperparathyroidism Often the result of benign tumors, this condition is caused by abnormally high levels of parathyroid hormones in the body. The symptoms may go unnoticed and include having too much calcium and/or phosphorus in the blood, too much hydrochloric acid in the stomach, kidney stones, weakened bones, and disrupted nerve function. Mild cases can be managed with medication; severe cases may require surgery to remove the parathyroid glands.

hyperthyroidism Any condition in which overactivity of the **thyroid gland** results in excessive levels of **thyroid hormone** in the body. It is diagnosed by measuring the levels of T_3, T_4, and TSH in the blood. Symptoms include nervousness; irritability; increased perspiration; thinning of the skin; fine, brittle hair; and muscular weakness, especially involving the upper arms and thighs. Your hands may shake and your heart may race. Your bowel movements may increase in frequency, though diarrhea is uncommon. Treatments include **antithyroid drugs,** destroying the gland (ablation) with radioactive iodine, and surgical removal of some or all of the thyroid gland (thyroidectomy). Hyperthyroidism is also called "thyrotoxicosis" and "overactive thyroid."

hypopituitarism Insufficient production of one, several, or all of the various hormones secreted by the pituitary gland, including **thyroid stimulating hormone (TSH).**

hypothalamus A small neuroendocrine gland in the brain near the pituitary. It secretes a number of stimulating and inhibiting hormones, including **thyrotropin-releasing hormone (TRH).** TRH stimulates **thyroid-stimulating hormone (TSH)**-secreting cells in the pituitary.

hypothyroidism An illness in which the amount of thyroid hormone in the body is below normal, resulting in a lowered metabolic rate and a general loss of vigor. Hypothyroidism is the most common thyroid abnormality—far more common than hyperthyroidism. Symptoms include feeling run down, slow, cold, tired, depressed, and disinterested in daily activities. Other symptoms may include dry and brittle hair, dry and itchy skin, constipation, muscle cramps, and, in women, increased menstrual flow.

iodine This element is an essential constituent of the **thyroid hormones** and is obtained from your diet. It is present in iodized salt, seafood, milk and other dairy products, and some vegetables (such as **kelp**). Insufficient dietary iodine can lead to hypothyroidism and goiter, especially in women.

isotope A variant form of an element with nearly identical chemical behavior but a slightly different atomic weight and electrical charge. Radioactive isotopes of iodine and technetium (a metallic element) are used in the treatment of some thyroid conditions.

isthmus A small band of thyroid tissue that crosses over the trachea (windpipe) and connects the left and right lobes of the thyroid gland.

kelp A dietary supplement made from the ashes of seaweed and used to provide **iodine.**

lymph gland (lymph node) The lymphatic system is similar to the circulatory system in that it is composed of vessels and transports fluid (lymph). Its main function is to neutralize bacteria and other pathogens. Thousands of small glands, also called **nodes,** are scattered throughout the vessels of the lymph system. The glands are where the activity of fighting bacteria takes place; during the fighting, the glands may become enlarged—inflamed and swollen. The most common areas in which this occurs are where there is a high concentration of glands—in the neck, under the arms, and in the groin. An enlarged lymph node in the neck is usually due to a sore throat but may be related to thyroid disease.

medullary-cell cancer A cancer of the medullary, C-, or parafollicular cells that lodge in the **thyroid gland** and secrete the hormone **calcitonin.**

multinodular goiter A goiter that contains many nodules. You may be **euthyroid** despite having multinodular goiter but may later become hyperthyroid or hypothyroid. Multinodular goiter is also called Plummer's disease.

myxedema A severe form of hypothyroidism characterized by thickened, stiff, swollen skin; dry skin and hair; and loss of mental and physical vigor. Left untreated, it can become critical and may result in coma or death. Myxedema is treated with **thyroid hormone replacement** drugs.

node The word literally means a knot, knob, swelling, or protuberance. Functionally, it describes a small, rounded organ or other bodily structure.

nodule A small node. (It may also be called a nodulus.)

nodule, cold See: Cold nodule.

nodule, hot See: Hot nodule.

nodulus See: Nodule.

oculomotor muscles The muscles that control eye movement. Their functionality may be impaired as a result of **hyperthyroidism,** which can cause eye pain, tearing, blurred or double vision, and reduced mobility, that is, you may have difficulty moving your eyes up and down or from side to side. This condition is called Graves' ophthalmopathy.

overactive thyroid See: Hyperthyroidism.

papillary carcinoma The most common form of thyroid cancer; papillary carcinoma is associated with radiation exposure and **hypothyroidism.** It spreads via the lymph system and typically is treated with some form of thyroidectomy. With small encapsulated tumors, surgery is almost always curative; with larger tumors, postoperative ablation of any remaining thyroid tissue with successive radioiodine treatments is advised. In either case, thyroid hormone replacement is given after surgery to reduce the possibility of regression of any remaining cancerous tissue and to prevent the symptoms of hypothyroidism.

parathyroid glands Four tiny glands located along the back and lower edge of the **thyroid gland.** These glands secrete parathyroid hormone, which controls the amount of calcium and phosphorous in your blood.

pituitary gland An endocrine gland embedded in the front of the brain. The pituitary gland secretes hormones that regulate a wide variety of body functions, including **thyroid stimulating hormone (TSH),** which is also known as thyrotropin.

Plummer's disease See: multinodular goiter.

radioactive iodine (RAI) Also called radioiodine, RAI is a generic term for one of the three isotopes of iodine used to treat or diagnose thyroid disorders. The isotope 131I is used to treat hyperthyroidism, thyroid cancer, and other thyroid disorders. Isotopes 123I and 132I are used for diagnostic tests.

radioiodine See: Radioactive iodine.

resin T₃ uptake This diagnostic test measures the amount of thyroid-binding globulin and other carrier proteins present in the blood. (The amount of protein available determines how much thyroid hormone can be bound.) The test helps to determine whether the total T_4 accurately reflects the concentration of free T_4, or if high or low amounts of the proteins are causing changes in the T_4 values.

reverse T₃ A biologically inactive form of triiodothyronine (T_3). Reverse T_3 is formed from normal T_3 and is identical to it except that the molecule is the mirror image of normal T_3.

Riedel's thyroiditis A very rare form of thyroid disease in which fibrous tissue causes the gland to harden and lose its ability to function. The fibrous tissue may extend out of the thyroid and press on the windpipe.

subacute viral thyroiditis See: De Quervain's thyroiditis.

subclinical hypothyroidism "Subclinical" describes a situation in which some biological disorder is present, but the typical symptoms of the illness have not arisen. Mildly increased or, as in the case of hypothyroidism, decreased levels of thyroid hormone often present subclinically. See also: Free T_3 test, free T_4 test, hyperparathyroidism.

suppurative thyroiditis An acute infection of the thyroid gland by micro-organisms that produce pus.

Synthroid The proprietary name of a medication used to treat hypothyroidism, goiter, and thyroid cancer, Synthroid is a manufactured version of the thyroid hormone thyroxine (T_4). See also: Thyroid-hormone replacement.

T₃ See: Triiodothyronine.

T₃-toxicosis Hyperthyroidism in which the level of **thyroid stimulating hormone (TSH)** is suppressed and the secretion of triiodothyronine (T_3) increases but the blood level of

thyroxine (T_4) remains constant. It may occur early in the course of **Graves' disease** or in association with a **hot nodule** in the **thyroid gland.**

T₄ See: Thyroxine.

TBG See: Thyroxine-binding globulin.

technetium See: Isotope.

thyroglobulin A protein that contains **iodine** and that the thyroid uses to make **thyroxine** (T_4) and **triiodothyronine** (T_3). Measuring blood levels of **thyroglobulin** helps determine whether any thyroid cells remain active after a total thyroidectomy or radioiodine ablation. The test also indicates if metastases have developed.

Thyroglobulin extracted from the thyroid glands of the Sus scrofa hog is a medication used to treat **hypothyroidism.**

thyroglobulin antibodies Thyroglobulin antibodies attack thyroglobulin stored in the **thyroid gland.** Higher than normal levels of thyroglobulin antibodies are suggestive of **Hashimoto's disease,** an autoimmune disease that leads to **hypothyroidism.** A more sensitive test measures microsomal (TPO) antibodies and is usually more accurate in establishing the diagnosis.

"thyroid" may also refer to a medicine derived from the cleaned, dried, and powdered thyroid gland of domesticated food animals (such as hogs).

thyroid crisis Sometimes called a "thyroid storm," this is a rare, but potentially fatal, episode of **hyperthyroidism.** Thyroid crisis usually occurs when someone with hyperthyroidism gets a second illness or infection, during withdrawal from antithyroid drugs, or after thyroid surgery. Its symptoms include fever, sweating, restlessness, racing heart rate (more than 100 beats a minute), irregular heart beat, congestive heart failure, and shock. The symptoms of shock include confusion, agitation, anxiety, and coma; panting, gasping, or abnormally fast breathing; fainting or feeling as if you would faint; and cool, clammy, or bluish (cyanotic) skin. NOTE: Thyroid crisis is a medical emergency, and immediate help should be obtained.

thyroid function test One of several diagnostic tests used to determine whether the thyroid is overactive (**hyperthyroidism**), underactive (**hypothyroidism**), or functioning normally (**euthyroid**). The most common—and reliable—of these tests is the **thyroid-stimulating hormone (TSH) test** with supersensitive assays.

thyroid gland An endocrine gland located at the pit of the throat that produces two hormones, **thyroxine (T₄)** and **triiodothyronine (T₃)**. These hormones help the thyroid gland regulate itself and also help the body convert food into energy and synthesize protein in all tissues.

thyroid hormone A general term for either or both of the hormones produced by the thyroid gland: **thyroxine (T₄)** and **triiodothyronine (T₃)**.

thyroid-hormone replacement A drug therapy that uses synthetic or organically derived versions of **triiodothyronine (T₃)** and **thyroxine (T₄)** to treat **hypothyroidism**. See also: Antithyroid drugs.

thyroid storm See: Thyroid crisis.

thyroidectomy The surgical removal of all or part of the thyroid gland. Removing the entire gland is called total thyroidectomy. Subtotal thyroidectomy is removing more than half, but less than all, of the gland. Thyroid lobectomy and hemithyroidectomy are names for surgeries in which only one lobe and the **isthmus** is excised. (The prefix *hemi-* means "half.")

thyroiditis Inflammation of the **thyroid gland** due to an **autoimmune disease** such as **Hashimoto's disease** or a virus, as with de **Quervain's thyroiditis**. The suffix *-itis* means "inflamed."

thyroid-stimulating antibodies These antibodies occupy the receptor sites on the surface of thyroid cells normally used by

thyroid- stimulating hormone (TSH). This makes the cells increase their secretion of thyroid hormone and leads to **hyperthyroidism.** The same antibody occurs temporarily in some **hypothyroid** patients who have a transient episode of hyperthyroidism. Thyroid-stimulating antibodies are sometimes called thyrotropin-receptor stimulating antibodies (TRS) or thyroid-stimulating immunoglobulins. See also: Graves' disease, Hashitoxicosis.

thyrotropin-receptor stimulating antibodies See: Thyroid-stimulating antibodies.

thyroid-stimulating immunoglobulins See: Thyroid-stimulating antibodies.

thyroid-stimulating hormone (TSH) Also called thyrotropin, TSH is a hormone secreted by the pituitary gland that stimulates the thyroid gland to produce **triiodothyronine (T₃)** and **thyroxine (T₄)**.

thyroid-stimulating hormone (TSH) test Measuring the amount of TSH helps determine **hypothyroidism** or **hyperthyroidism.** This test is more sensitive than the thyrotropin-releasing hormone (TRH) test and is commonly used in place of it. Low TSH levels are not necessarily an indication of thyroid disease; the secretion of TSH may be temporarily reduced by nonthyroidal illnesses, either physical or psychiatric, or during the first three months of a pregnancy.

thyrotoxicosis See: Hyperthyroidism.

thyrotropin See: Thyroid-stimulating hormone (TSH).

thyrotropin-receptor stimulating immunoglobulins See: Thyroid-stimulating antibodies.

thyrotropin-releasing hormone (TRH) A hormone secreted by the **hypothalamus** that stimulates the pituitary to secrete **thyroid-stimulating hormone (TSH)**.

thyrotropin-releasing hormone test A diagnostic test used to measure the amount of **thyroid-stimulating hormone (TSH)** secreted into the blood in reaction to an injection of synthetic TRH. This test has largely been superseded by the thyroid-stimulating hormone test.

thyroxine One of the hormones produced by the **thyroid gland.** Thyroxine contains four iodine atoms and is often called T_4. It helps the body convert food into energy and synthesize protein in all tissues. Synthetic and organically derived thyroxine is used to treat hypothyroidism.

thyroxine-binding globulin (TBG) Globulin is one of three proteins that **thyroxine (T_4)** binds to in order to be carried through the bloodstream. The others are prealbumin and albumin, but globulin carries about 70 percent of the hormone. When the TBG level is low, the levels of total T_4 and total T_3 are also low because their main carrier protein is reduced. When the TBG is high, the levels of total T_4 and total T_3 are raised. A thyroid function test measures the TBG levels in the blood and relies on the **free thyroxine index** to relate them to the total T_3 and total T_4 levels. However, because the bound hormone is biologically inactive, high or low levels of TBG do not necessarily indicate thyroid disorder. If your levels of thyroid-stimulating hormone (TSH), free T_4, and free T_3 are normal, you will be **euthyroid.**

total T_3 test A thyroid function test that measures the concentration of bound and free **triiodothyronine (T_3)** in the blood. Because 99.5 percent of the hormone is bound to carrier proteins such as thyroid-binding globulin (TBG), anything that raises or lowers the concentration of these proteins in the blood will similarly raise or lower the total T_3.

total T_4 test A thyroid function test that measures the concentrations of bound and free **thyroxine (T_4)** in the blood. Because 99.5% of the hormone is bound to carrier proteins, such as thyroid-binding globulin (TBG), anything that raises or lowers the concentration of the proteins in the blood will similarly raise or lower the total T_4.

TRH See: Thyrotropin-releasing hormone.

TRH test See: Thyrotropin-releasing hormone test.

triiodothyronine Also known as T_3, this is one of the two thyroid hormones. It is an iodine-containing hormone derived from thyroxine and helps the thyroid to regulate itself.

TSH See: Thyroid-stimulating hormone.

TSH test *See*: Thyroid-stimulating hormone test.

viral thyroiditis See: de Quervain's thyroiditis.

Index